AWAKE ATHLETE

WHEN MASTERY IS YOUR ONLY OPTION

JESS GUMKOWSKI

A YOGITRIATHLETE PRODUCTION

To Mary,

I am forever grateful to you for teaching me the hardest lessons
of my life and serving as an inspiration to finish this book.

In the face of intense resistance and unprecedented trauma,
I felt your reminders from beyond to finish what I started.

You are forever a beam of light, a divine messenger,
a generous provider and my masterful teacher.

The message you dreamed of sharing with the world is here.
You would have loved this book.

Awake and ready.

Mary Knott
*Spiritual Aspirant, Ultra Endurance Athlete, Veterinarian,
Daughter, Sister, Friend*
1976—2021

Acknowledgements

As I never wrote a word in this book with ownership of one single letter, I owe eternal thanks to the stream of infinite intelligence for allowing me to be the steward of what lies before you.

From a worldly perspective, several people and one particularly handsome canine played significant roles in bringing this book into physical manifestation.

My first person of recognition is my husband, BJ. For all the dinners you cooked and the coffee you brewed, the countless times you brought me the power cord to my computer and did not interrupt me when I said I was "going in," I would be years behind in this creation without you. From early in our relationship, your unshakeable belief that I was to write a book, or books as you say, kept the spark flamed for decades.

To my mom, Joan Costello, I am beholden to you for birthing me, loving me, and living the example of a life steeped in trust and strength. My whole life, I've been asked about my strong mindset; it is you who poured the foundation of my beliefs that are the breadth of this book.

My dad, Lou Costello, for showing me the steady way through life's challenges and never giving up simply because something is hard, like the monumental task of writing a book. Semper fi, dear soldier.

My sister Susanne Goldstein, your unwavering belief in me deeply informs my ability to finish what I start. I am forever grateful to you for mirroring my greatness and always having something sparkly for me to wear.

My brother Matthew Costello, someone I feel a very ancient connection with and who never questions my capability to conquer anything I set out to do. I see you in your power Matty, and it fueled me to complete this book.

To Teri Gumkowski, you were an angel on this earth for a time and my mother-in-law. You left me with an undying mission to love without condition, which strengthened the messages in this book.

To my sweetest boy, Clark, your existence in this life reminds me of the trust and unconditional love that allows for joy. Thank you for lying by my side, eating the tops of my strawberries, and being my unfailing compatriot while writing this book.

To Bob Arnold, my spiritual teacher who is only interested in diving into the deep end, I would have remained lost without you. Your acceptance of me is as profound as your belief that I am one of the 1%. I look forward to learning from you in future lifetimes but hopefully, not too many more on this earth.

To my yoga teachers, Philip Urso and Renee Deslauriers, your earth-fire combination supported me to no end, called for the death of my ignorance, and heavily influenced the stream of knowledge that flows within these pages.

To Tara Calhiman, Goldyn Duffy, and Liz McHutcheon, fist pumps and namastes to the three of you for braving through the earliest version of these pages with kindness and optimism. Your open hearts, white gloves, and constructive feedback impacted this final product. I am grateful.

To Valerie Griffiths and Meghan Leighton, the air and earth that offer me balance. Thank you for being prominent believers that it is time for the world of sports to meet Awake Athlete. I finally know what I have seen others experience; a sisterhood of divine proportion. I bow to you both.

And to the YogiTriathlete and Awake Athlete communities, you are the dream come true; this is for you.

"What's the use of doing anything that's too easy?
Anybody can do it.
The glory comes only when you do something others can't
easily do."

Swami Satchidananda
Yoga Master

Contents

INTRODUCTION

"You may go on reading any number of books on Meditation. They can only tell you 'Realize the Self'. The Self cannot be found in books. You have to find it for yourself in yourself."

Ramana Maharshi

It was the spring of 2020 when it all began to move through me at a fierce pace.

The world had shut down within days due to the pandemic, and in the halting of that momentum, I followed an inner directive to slow down and go deeper into my meditation and mindful practices. I stopped waking up to an alarm. Instead, I allowed my body to wake up naturally, and I returned to my yoga mat daily with a higher level of devotion. I sat for meditation twice a day without fail, and it wasn't long before I tapped into a stream of intelligibility which I quickly harnessed as the entity Awake Athlete.

I began writing, and the stream fed me. Within a month, I knew I had something much more extensive, but it would take time. However, I also knew the information needed to be released as soon as possible. After being the host of the YogiTriathlete podcast for years, it felt natural and exciting to get this knowledge into the world through podcasting. And so, amid quarantine, I climbed into a small closet in the loft I share with my husband, BJ, and dog, Clark, and hit record. The first season of the Awake Athlete podcast, with 14 short-form episodes designed for binging, dropped to the world in August 2020. Seasons two and three followed in consecutive years.

As I sit here now, in late summer of 2022, dotting many *i's* and crossing a ton of *t's* in the final stages of this manuscript, season four of the podcast is also steadily taking form. Where it will end is anyone's guess. All I know is that as long as the information flows, I am grateful to be its bridge to the physical world. Becoming this bridge is a lifelong journey of waking up, and for you to understand this book and the wellspring from which it came, you must first meet my friend. I refer to her as *she*, but it may be a *he* or *they* in your world. That is entirely up to you. The only thing that matters to me is that she is a friend that you befriend by the time you turn the last page of this book.

So let me start by saying she is an old friend of mine, the "pick-up where we left off" kind of friend; no guilt trips or expectations. She simply waits with eternal patience for my return. She is loyal, better than a golden retriever, and not just to me. She is a steadfast comrade to anyone who takes a chance on her. She does, however, tend to disrupt my plan. This can make me frustrated, but not with her. It is never her but myself that I cannot tolerate. During those times, she holds me with neutrality and compassion despite my inability to do the same.

This friend of mine, we sit together every day now. The days of skipping my visits with her are no more. I have seen a day in my life without her and no longer desire to live that way. Her loving embrace is vast, and it is seemingly never-ending. I rely sincerely on her power as the storms in my mind rain down and the skies open to purge my greatest enemy. She is impenetrable in the wake of my humanness. I feel her smile as I sometimes lean my weight into her and shed tears of profound sadness. When I cannot find my way on my own, she leads me back to expansion so I may breathe again. She holds my hand as I judge myself and indulge in irrelevant thoughts that pull my attention away from her. She brings me to my knees with her dispassion which reminds me, time and again, that this is my journey, and I am the only one who can walk it. No one is here to save me, especially her.

I have realized my Self, and through this reacquaintance, I get to save my future from great sorrow. She warms me as my body falls still into moments of complete connectedness and assures me from deep within that this is truly my home. She helps me stand when I feel my legs will crumble and, as she deems me ready, gives me the full load to bear.

Day after day, we meet, some days begrudgingly, but alas, I knock at her door. No matter the time of day, weather, or any other factor, she always meets me in the same fashion, utter acceptance. Somedays, I feel myself vaporize into her everythingness within the first few moments of our reunion, while on other days, our interaction is the great battle of my life.

Our friendship grows, and I trust her implicitly, as I have since I heard her speak to me as a young child. I know that I am listening, and her ways are sinking in because my heart is opening to the world exactly as it is, without any need for change. She has given me eyes to see myself in others. She has taught me to pause so that I may choose away from darkness, and she has shown me that even in the most intense moments of life, when I suffocate in the prison of my body, I always have a breath to breathe. I know what love is now, and I am embody selflessness more each day because of our time together. She has done nothing, yet her inaction is what drives me further on my path.

We no longer just meet in the mornings; she is always with me. I see her in my dreams, where I ask for the messages I am to receive. At the end of each day, I lay it all down in her honor because I am clear now that it was never mine. I wake up each moment because of her and celebrate every awakening with her. Then, on the days when it seems too much, and I hide in the protective cocoon of my home, I sit as tall as I can and close my eyes to rest in her loving arms again. It is here that I connect with my never-ending Self, the part of me that is always home and the one who craves the difficult moments because it knows they are the reason I am here.

She is the dearest friend I have ever known and the one I pray
for all to know. She is the facilitator of modern-day warriors
who will shift the world from hate to love and from separate
to one as they awaken to their truth. She is the gateway to our
extraordinary power and the end of suffering as we know it.
She is a masterful mentor to all who endeavor her technique;
she is meditation.

Throughout the pages of this book, you will repeatedly hear
about meditation because it is the base of all that I practice,
and teach on the path to mastery which I am walking just like
you. Without a steadfast meditation practice rooted in stillness,
the techniques and perspectives I offer in this book will only
supply temporary relief from the human condition and fleeting
glimpses of a masterful life. Neither of which is a waste, by
no means. Everything is a seed planted. But meditation as
the primary tool for training the mind is far superior to any
other method, yet it supports all other techniques in yielding
maximum benefit.

Meditation is an unparalleled accelerator for anyone who
feels there is something higher to achieve in life. It teaches us
to watch our thoughts and learn where our minds dwell. It
provides an education into our minds' tendencies, allowing us
to overcome what is holding us back in the performance of life.

Committing to a sitting practice inserts a regular break into
the addiction to always be doing and attunes us to a higher
perspective from which we can see ourselves and the world
with new eyes. This is awakening. It is freedom from our

identification with maya, the cosmic illusion of what appears to be real and true. It is the dream of being separate that makes us see multiplicity when there is only one. Maya holds an inherent denial of our interconnectivity and the creative power we maintain to achieve anything we set our minds to. The spark that guided you to pick up this book is the awakening spark; it's a sure sign that your higher mind is signaling you to be a more prominent player in how you move through the world.

When you finish this book, you will know when you are reacting to life with an old worldview and you will have techniques at the ready to shift your mindset. You will also have tools to traverse trauma in an awakened state and to utilize breath's simplicity as a flawless and timeless tool. You will have recipes for success, mantras for concentration, and an enlightened take on performance. And whether or not you identify as an athlete, I hope you will see that this book is for everyone because our inherent right to move from servantry to mastery is not just for those who line up on a start line. Awake Athlete is for all who breathe this breath of life and live within the vehicle of a body.

And so now, let's you and I venture together on a journey that I intend will forever shift your mind. I am thrilled to invite you to embody a mindset like nothing we have seen before in the world of sports. I implicitly trust the purpose of this book to serve those who are ready for the grand awakening of their life. The world has never seen a book like Awake Athlete, but it has come time for you and me to step onto the precipice of true greatness through mind mastery and set it as the new and exceptional norm.

CHAPTER ONE

EVOLUTION OF AN AWAKE ATHLETE

"Most of our troubles are due to passionate desire for and
attachment to things that we misapprehend as enduring entities."

His Holiness the 14th Dalai Lama

It was cooler than a typical evening in McLeod Ganj, a suburb of Dharamsala, India. We gathered around a series of small tables under a clear sky at the outdoor cafe. This night was one of the few on which we could make out the high peaks of the Himalayas, the clouds moving about within the last light of the day. I was 37 years old and in a hillside village, 4,700 feet above sea level, double that in miles away from home, a half-day journey to the nearest industrialized city, and in the company of Tibetan refugees whose lives somehow seemed better than mine.

In moments like these, I feel the magic of life. It can be hard to comprehend how I get there, but then I remember an understanding I have always carried; every moment in life builds upon the next. So it's never one decision but a lifetime or lifetimes of them that gets us to where we are in a moment. And that night, I remember leaning back in my chair and feeling blessed for all I have lived and traversed because it led me to that cafe in India, an international journey that served as a great awakening in my life.

As I recall, there were six of us that night; four female students and two teachers, myself, and my friend Louise, a fellow massage therapist and instructor from the Boulder College of Massage Therapy (BCMT). We were several days into our trip, and the familiarity among our group was evident. Laughter was always on the menu with these joyous women even when they told inside jokes, clearly about us, in their native Tibetan tongue.

I fixated on the women as they shared their stories and spread their happiness generously. I kept tasting the air and feeling my feet in my shoes. I wanted to be in the moment like never before. I was learning about happiness in simplicity. It was novel to me. I suppose I didn't think it was possible to be so without *all the stuff*. I gained an understanding of their courageous escape to Dharamsala from their homeland of Tibet and more about the Tibetan uprising in March of 1959 that cost tens of thousands of Tibetan lives at the hands of the Chinese military. I learned that it had been a half-century since the Dalai Lama's escape from Tibet and the establishment of the Tibetan government-in-exile.

I asked the women what message I should bring home to the

United States. How did they want us to support and raise awareness of Tibetan culture? They told me not to be bitter or talk poorly about the Chinese government or its people. They said China was confused and scared, which is why they did what they did. There was no need to punish them. They asked me to forgive if I was angry and be compassionate towards those who carried out such wrongdoings because karmic repayment was inevitable. There was neutrality in their tone and an absence of the vengeful satisfaction one could expect or justify. I felt a knowingness from within to heed the guidance; it carried a power I had been familiar with throughout my life.

It was in early 2009 when this opportunity to teach massage to Tibetan refugees in India came to my awareness. The trip was set for September that year, and there was no debate for me. I knew I was going from the moment I caught the first wind of the news. I had known for years that I would take big trips in my life, and these knowings always carried innate patience. I knew I would be ready to say "yes" when the time came. This was one of those times. I noticed that my ego also liked the idea very much. The praise of doing something so noble was too good to turn down. A part of me could not wait to climb onto a pedestal and share the news, which I did time and again. I was not awake to the ego back then as I am now, so yes, I used this trip to seek selfish praise, but that never overrode my grateful heart.

The trip was the brainchild of my friend Carol, one of my earliest mentors in living a creative life freely without succumbing to the engrained demands of society. She is a renegade to this day. At the time, she was the Director of Student Affairs at BCMT, where I worked part-time in the marketing department, a job I obtained after attending BCMT's extensive program to become a massage therapist. Being involved with the school professionally and working as a practitioner in the healing arts was beginning to shift my life radically. I was growing closer to something I always craved, a more meaningful existence.

In preparation for the trip, I learned more about the refugees we would be teaching and the town where we'd be staying. There was so much I did not know about Tibet and the strife its people endured. I did not realize that children walked through the Himalayas in handmade slippers under the guidance of warriors paid by their parents to get them to safety. I did not know that it was not only for their shot at a future but also for the Tibetan culture's preservation.

I grew up in Sandwich, Massachusetts, the oldest town on Cape Cod and the hometown of American author Thornton W. Burgess. A small village where "Free Tibet" bumper stickers on high-priced SUVs were the extent of my Tibetan education. I realized that I never had to consider my role in cultural preservation. I felt ignorant and a little angry, but simultaneously, I was open to absorbing the truth of what I was learning without judging the life I was born into.

I do not believe there is luck in this life, and I do not feel lucky because I grew up on Cape Cod. I am deeply grateful, of course, but I understand that the ebb and flow of my life are unique to my soul journey. Just as the students I was about to teach in India were living circumstances unique to their soul journeys. Through my spiritual studies, I now understand that all beings incarnate into the exact circumstances that allow for that soul's most extraordinary evolution. And although I know our essence to be the same, our worldly existence differs greatly. I wish I could agree that all are born equal, but I cannot. What I do agree with is the wisdom of the sages that proclaim every human being has the opportunity to wake up in this life.

For my story and alignment in this existence, the environment of my primary years did not lend much diversity to my upbringing, but I'm not sure that matters because I grew up in a home that taught me to love all. And isn't that the ultimate teaching? Actually, the complete teaching was I did not have to like everyone, but I must love all. My mom and dad are faithful and fiery, so it was love and forgiveness, but also, it was not putting up with crap from anyone.

It is true; I have lived an incredibly abundant life. I am deeply loved and was raised under guiding principles such as presence and gratitude. Sure, my family experienced financial stress, and I saw my dad get laid off more than once. But despite the challenges we faced, my parents always found a way. I saw my mom return to work full-time and become the breadwinner she remains today, close to her 90s (and crushing it)!

Our home was spacious and comfortable. We lived in a custom-built colonial in Jacob's Farm, a coveted neighborhood for its time. I was never without food, a roof, clothing, or accessories. Oh, if you could have seen my accessory collection. I lived in plenty, that is true, but I also believed in lack. I worried about money and battled with not feeling enough, yet there was no evidence of lack in my life. All I had ever known were Cape Cod problems, and I was on the verge of a remote stay in a developing nation. There was so much unknown ahead, and I was as scared as I was excited. Admittedly, I was craving it, I was restless and hungry for a courageous quest at this point in my life. There was a part of me that was choking on the comfort of my day in and day out. I wanted to experience life through new eyes. A pulsation in my heart rose through layers of conditioning, calling me to flame a spark of adventure. I needed this experience for my next level of growth, and I knew it. My thirst for knowledge called for quenching, and all of it was me already walking the spiritual path. It's the same path you are on, the one you have traversed for an eternity already. The one we can never fall off because, at our core, we are spiritual beings.

Anticipation built for months. The program was named Massage For Peace. We were scheduled to teach for seven days at Lha Charitable Trust in McCleod Ganj, and we set out to raise money to cover the cost of our travels and make a hefty cash donation for Lha's future programming. It was a brilliant and perfect plan because it was service work, something I wanted more of. Admittedly though, I still carried a selfish disposition which I discovered was rooted in competitiveness so natural to me I couldn't even see it. I just thought everyone wanted to win at everything and be the best all the time. But, after an uproar from my BCMT classmates when I stated I didn't have a competitive bone in my body, I realized that being competitive was a characteristic of my unique make-up. One that needed more proper channeling because sometimes it was hurtful to others. This was when I turned to triathlon; unbeknownst to me, the channel to Awake Athlete also opened.

My competitive tendencies did not extinguish during massage school, and in the case of triathlon, they were thriving. I continued to be driven by them, but it began to shift towards the betterment of others, not just the betterment of me. At my BCMT graduation, I was awarded the community service award, which was my first big taste of giving of myself to others. It was a new type of satisfaction, but the high number of service hours also came from wanting to win every award available and graduate at the top of my class. I have always felt a strong drive to excel, and I don't believe anything is wrong with that drive. It is who I am in this life, and maybe you can relate. We athletes share this and it is our most powerful tool for staying the course to mastery and living awake.

My experience at BCMT, first as a student and then as a team member, was a big waking-up time in my life and this trip to India was a natural extension of that growth. I was beginning to understand the layers and burdens I carried through the many heart-opening practices I engaged in throughout my massage therapy education. For example, non-violent communication and embodied knowledge of the subtle energy body, or as scientists call it, the biofield[1]. A concept that woke

1 The biofield is a field of energy that surrounds the body and extends out about eight feet from the gross physical body, it cannot be seen but it can be felt and measured.

me up to a curiosity that perhaps I am more than just flesh. I began to worry less about the world's circumstances as I gained more wisdom about universal laws like the law of attraction and realized that perhaps the change I desired to see in the world began with me. I recognized that I didn't need to carry so much on my shoulders. As I leaned into healing modalities like acupuncture and energy work, I naturally moved toward the vulnerability necessary to let go of the pain I carried. With that, I noticed a growing desire for a simpler life overall.

It was the life I had heard about but doubted for so many years; you know, the one where happiness comes from the inside. A lesson our Tibetan students and the people of India showed me throughout our visit; minor amounts of material with persistent feelings of happiness. And that evening at the cafe, I shared with our students how impressed Louise and I were with their ability to pick up the massage techniques quickly. Day after day, we shook our heads in disbelief as the students demonstrated basic and advanced techniques with natural ability and quality of touch akin to years of experience. The women smiled in response to my observance as if they knew something we did not, which was apparent almost every time we spoke.

"Our minds are clear. They are not cluttered like American minds", said Tashi. She spoke with an energy that was as light as a feather, causing me to reflect. I never thought of my mind as cluttered; I never examined my mind at all. Up until then, I allowed it to be what it was, and it was my master.

These women had plenty of reasons to have clutter in their

minds. It wasn't as if they had not been exposed to intense
life experiences. I mean, they left their families and walked a
deathly route through the Himalayas. They lost members of
their group along the way and were almost captured by Nepali
police more than once. But somehow, they were not clouded
with the trauma of their history. The reality of their past did
not weigh them down. They had moved on and moved forward
while not denying what had transpired. I saw something that
evening I had not seen before. I didn't have words for it, but
now I do. It was detachment accompanied by loving-kindness.
It was the powerful neutrality that I have come to know as
unconditional love.

In *The Yoga Sutras of Patanjali*[2], it is written that life is a passing
show, and to cling to one instant creates tension in life. As
Tibetan Buddhists, these women were raised within a construct
of detachment. A conscious life of forgiveness and letting go,
one that prepared them to say goodbye to their families and
lose their homeland. A homeland most likely never believed
to be theirs in the first place. I imagine they thought it was
nobody's land and yet every being's land.

Over the remainder of our days together, I learned more about
detachment and the freedom it lends to its practitioner. Some
people hear detachment and think of apathy or complacency,
but that is not the case. These students cared very much about
what they were learning, but they weren't getting caught up

---

2 The yoga sutras are a collection of 196 verses that guides one to attain self-realization through
the study and practice of yoga, the science of the mind. Self-realization is the attainment of one's
full potential; realization of the true Self. The version I study is translated by Sri Swami
Satchinanda who is one of the most revered yoga masters of our time and also my guru's guru.

in the complications of a cluttered mind or the tension experienced when we cling. They detached from the massage stroke, their thoughts about the stroke, the outcome of their efforts, and the traumas of their past. Detachment gave them presence, a clear and constant stream of precious moments linked within a lifetime. Moments devoid of time and free of the ego.

People live with immense stress levels in our modern society because they are attached to outcomes. We are worried about what will be and how the results will play out. If we work hard enough, this attachment path does work, but it is heavy and slow. It enhances doubt and worry, both of which clutter the hallways of our minds and dull our ability to perform at our best.

Through the quality of humility, I saw a way of life in India that was easeful and powerful. I had difficulty comprehending such meekness, not to mention compassion, but I was learning more every day. I honored their wishes and took note of their wisdom on happiness, but nothing shifted my life more than Tashi's take on the cluttered mind and the connection I made to allowing life to pass without tension. I walked away from that conversation with a strong desire to live within the flow of giving and receiving, letting go and moving forward. I wanted nothing to stand in my way of being better.

The Bhagavad Gita[3] teaches that utter detachment and unwavering devotion are the qualities necessary to win the only war we must wage in this life. The war within. The one that Tashi and her fellow students were living every day with a level of grace I had not witnessed prior. They had every reason to choose a life of grievance, but instead, they lived for the moment because they knew, without being scared, that any day may be their last. They hold life with reverence and are awake without emotion to the karma, or cause and effect, that mapped the story of their life thus far.

To say that evening in Dharamsala launched my spiritual journey is false, but most assuredly, it catapulted me into the next level of spiritual living. I have felt a power deep inside me for as long as I can remember. It is below my heart and burns like the ball of fire in our sky. Like most of you, I grew up in a world that believed in separation, I was taught to work hard because that's the only way anything will be worthwhile. I considered no other way. I used my will to make things happen and often disregarded the feelings of others. I worked hard until burnout then I fought rest even when my body showed me glaring signs that it needed rest. I repeated cycles that compounded exhaustion in my body and mind.

My experience in India showed me a new way to direct my will. One that benefits the good of all and includes ease through letting go of the clutter in my mind. Surrendering to

3 *Bhagavad Gita* is a 700-verse Hindu scripture often referred to as the Gita. It is a poem known as the "Song of The Lord" composed by an ancient sage named Krishna Dvaipayana Vyasa. It presents the everyman's battle with the mind. The battle we all must wage in order to truly know who we are in this life. Through the experience of Arjuna, the greatest warrior of all time and his charioteer, Krishna, the student learns mind mastery through practices such as meditation, devotion and detachment. It takes place on a battlefield and is a part of the epic Mahabharata which details the struggle between two groups of family, the Kauravas and the Pandavas, during the Kurukshetra War.

the truth of suffering in this world but not carrying it all on my shoulders. It was a concept that never really occurred to me before. I knew there were people dedicated to serving others, Mother Teresa, Sally Struthers, and Lady Diana. I grew up watching those figures advocate for others, but I just thought that was for them, not for me. I had zero notion that my energy, and yours too, affect the collective of all beings in every moment or that if hard work is the only way to achieve, I will not succeed by any other means than hard work.

When I returned home from India, I held a clear vision of my continued growth, and there was something about me that was less burdened. I self-regulated enough to realize that I still loved my Livingston entry bench from Pottery Barn, but I did go on to live from a higher perspective and expanded view.

Just one year later, my husband BJ and I left Boulder, Colorado, and moved back to Newport, Rhode Island, where we had met and fallen in love more than a decade before. Shortly after settling into our new home, I met my meditation teacher, or as I call him, Meditator Bob (MB). Then a few months later, my yoga mentor, Philip. These two men offered me tools to accelerate my path to enlightenment and humbled me greatly in recognition of my ego. I once heard Sailesh Rao of the organization Climate Healers describe enlightenment as the ability to experience the world as it is without judgment. Or, as MB tells me often, "be okay with whatever it is."

So yeah, I'm not enlightened yet, but I have the tools and knowledge, and when you finish this book, so will you. This guide shines a light on the mechanisms of the ego and the clutter of the conditioned mind. It gives you the tools to be the master of those things and the knowledge to see that your highest potential in sport and life is at your disposal right now. It reveals the purpose of this world and the darkness that exists in contrast to its light.

The teachings I share in the coming pages are primarily from yoga practices and my interpretation of yogic wisdom. The base for all the inner work I discuss is the discipline of meditation. Regular practice of stillness is the foundation, not the add-on. For me, meditation became a non-negotiable pretty quickly once I committed to sit. Even though the first year was a slug-fest, I used my will to remain consistent. Maybe it will be natural for you, and you'll be like one of those athletes who qualify for a championship at their first triathlon. Either way, the awake athlete path yields irrevocable shifts that lead to free indulgence in the joys of athletic adventure. It is a path that awakens us to the incredible power and truth of our nature while utilizing our endurance endeavors as vehicles to master our minds and win the war within.

So please, know that you have stepped onto a pathway of excellence that very few will consider in their lifetime. Most people will not buy it; they will chalk it up to new age woo-woo or give it a shot only to fall victim to the lies of their untrained minds. Most will settle for mediocre instead of the miraculous because they believe the miraculous is something out of the ordinary instead of an experience readily available each day.

As you read on, keep the following rule in the forefront of your experience, take what resonates and leave the rest. Use what you do not agree with to define what you do agree with and desire. And above all else, live the life you desire and be very stubborn about it. The laws of magnetism are real, and there are only two ways to live this life, as a deliberate creator or someone who lives by default. Either awake or asleep, the choice is yours. What we focus on expands, like attracts like; every action has an equal and opposite reaction. These are laws of science defined thousands of years ago by the yogis and confirmed in recent centuries by material scientists.

We live in a world of untrained minds. We mire in the minutia, focus on the negative, get stuck in the problem, overcomplicate meaning, and get trapped in trying. We miss what we are ready to put into action because we lack focus, so we ignore the teachings of a moment. We fall victim to the model of society which reveres the intellect and denies the spirit. We read books, attend conferences and talk our faces off about what we will start on Monday, but that is not how change occurs. We evolve only through experience by putting the knowledge we acquire into action; otherwise, the intellect becomes a waste of space. Applying the principles of yoga throughout our life positions us in harmony with universal law and the power of our essence. This is not how most people live; this is how the 1% live.

I consider those students in India a part of the 1%, for I had never received such insight as I did during that trip. The wisdom they shared with me during our short time together woke me up to a new way of seeing the world; its joys and horrors, my joys and horrors. The entire experience was a massive awakening for me. When I boarded the plane to Delhi in September 2009, I thought I was on a mission to bring peace through massage to refugees who needed it, as if they were in lack of it. I never considered that it was I who was in need. This experience set a new course for my life, leading me to where I sit now.

From time to time, I think about that night at the cafe and the hundreds of other moments shared in sacred communion with souls I was destined to meet on the other side of the globe. They showed me a new way to be and their wisdom remains strong within me still today.

In reading this book, I hope you become inspired to live against the grain alongside me. A way of being that allows you to stand with surefootedness and nullify doubt when all physical evidence reveals reasons to doubt. And I hope you seek the truth of what lies underneath the tiniest subatomic particle known to man living inside you right now. Because I know, if you do, you will discover the truth of what moves your breath and beats your heart. It is the one unchanging force in a universe that is always changing, the river of boundless energy that is you.

MB told me once that there are many doors in but only one door out. So, however your path gets you here, whenever you get here, and whoever you are here, know that you are right on time because it's this moment. The only one that will ever matter. This one, right now.

CHAPTER TWO

BE THE ONE IN THOUSANDS

"Step into the fire of self-discovery.
This fire will not burn you.
It will only burn what you are not."

Mooji

We are athletes. We have the desire for far-reaching goals and the innate tools to master them. We put in the work, we always have, and strive to go beyond what is reasonable most days of the week because that feels normal to us. Our lives do not exhaust us because the fire of our desire burns steadfastly from deep within. We are a unique breed. Determined, driven, and focused by our nature. We see something, we set a goal, and we attain it. Some of us have been athletes for as long as we can remember, while others are just beginning to realize their attunement towards an athletically driven life. We pride ourselves on eating hills for breakfast, and we live and breathe discipline. We challenge ourselves regularly in our training and crave more because we know that is how we grow.

We have already evolved beyond the norm and will continue to advance because life is a net gain journey that moves us all forward. There is nothing we can do that will lead us astray from our path, and over time, no matter what, we will all develop a driving desire to know higher states of truth. Since this book is in your hands, I presume you are there now, and to your relevant readiness, you are here to wake up to something more. It may be a pull that you are feeling but cannot yet describe. I know you are here because you are interested in training your mind, yet I wonder if you know how deep we will go?

The truth is, despite what brought you here and what you hope to take away, most of you will not stick on the path of training the mind in the ways I offer in this book. You will go far, no doubt. You will go further than most on this earth, but only one out of 1,000 says MB will go the distance. One out of thousands, states the Gita, will attain self-mastery over the mind and live an awakened reality. I know I am one out of thousands. It is that power I told you about, the one I've been deeply connected to my entire life, that tells me so. And, with over seven billion people on this planet, plenty of you are also one in thousands.

We athletes are tailor-made to wake up and train our minds because we are already disciplined and dedicated. These two qualities that allow us to excel in sports are the same that allow us to excel in mental training. It takes a high level of repetitive practice to achieve mind mastery, but most of you are already doing this in your physical training. I'm simply inviting you to take these natural strengths into your mental training. Applying your athlete spirit to a regular meditation practice, along with the practical application of the techniques and perspectives offered in this book, will make your training program complete.

We take the roof off our limitations when we entertain new viewpoints and question the mind chatter that leaves us feeling sub-par. And this is the beginning of freedom. From here, we step into an advanced way of doing things and embrace the understanding that we came here to experience joy, not as a fleeting emotion but as a state of being. Unaffected by external circumstances, it is a steady state for traversing life. One that is acquired by putting knowledge into action. We cannot intellectualize ourselves into expansion. Understanding or reading about an awakened life is not equivalent to living an awakened life. As we become more present through mindful practice, we see that training the mind is something we can do in every moment. As a result, mind mastery becomes a way of life.

The path of the awake athlete is a bold relaxation into the arms of something greater and waking up to see that you are of the very same essence. This may sound extreme, but all you need to do now is stay open. Open to the existence of a 10,000-foot view of life that is zoomed out and forward thinking. Open to expanding your mind and changing your brain. Open to allowing all that keeps you small to fall away and open to a life that you do not fully know yet. There is clutter in the hallways of our minds; this is for certain, but what is also certain is our right to be free of it.

As a result of waking up through meditation and mindful living, we turn up the volume of the seemingly silent voice of our truth and calibrate ourselves to excellence. It is not a four-step plan or a seven-minute workout; it is experience in its purest form. It's a practice you will practice for the rest of your time here on earth. It's the ultimate ultra, the extremest endurance event you will ever know, and the most extraordinary battle you will ever want to fight.

If you take this leap and go all-in, you will encounter more bliss, power, and calm beyond anything you have experienced before in this life. An unfettered perfection will permeate every facet of your being with a high degree of merit and efficiency. Every relationship in your life will improve, none more so than the one with yourself. You will face every single one of your fears along the way, I promise you will, but you will learn to look at every aspect of them and see them in truth. And if you stay the course and practice what you learn, you will stop indulging the mind's addiction to making big deals out of small things, and the space and peace you desire will arise.

Along the way, it is inevitable that the demands of the intellect will fool some of you burgeoning awake athletes as it grows impatient with the lack of tangible results after so many months or even days. And in the company of such mental noise, most will choose to doze off back into life because good enough feels like enough. Their ego will fight tooth and nail over the concept that doing nothing changes everything. And most will be too scared to step into a life of possibility because the mind is their master, and fear of the unknown has become their reality.

Those of you who remain steadfast and awaken to the layers that cloud the truth will see realities within your thought life that keep you from the very thing you are working so hard to achieve. It's okay; all of us who have walked before you have seen the same. But, I can tell you that over time, within a commitment to know yourself well, these layers lose their power, and your continued practice renders them mute because all untruths eventually burn away.

For me, living awake has wholly diminished my unconscious belief in lack. And even though I am often tested and challenged with unhelpful thoughts of not being enough or the fallacy that I won't ever have enough money, I can starve those thoughts of my attention now because I know that there is only abundance in this universe and I get to choose the flavor of my abundance. Because we live in a world that leans towards the negative, we tend to choose an abundance of precisely what we do not want. Unfortunately, many choose to live with an abundance of anger or sadness, financial lack, and low self-worth. I have done the same and can see that these unconscious choices kept me prisoner from a higher, freer expression. If you stay the course, you too will awaken to such lies and eventually be free from them as you train your mind to stop energizing them into your reality.

To succeed in this, we must let go of the belief that we need to make anything happen; where you are right now is the perfect jumping-off point for all you desire. Let go of any agenda that you meditate to get something, and know that lightening up your grip on the wheel of life will attune you quicker to the inner calm that is your invincibility. It is surrender that I am eluding to, and it is essential on this path to discovering ease within growth opportunities. We will encounter challenges in times of growth and change. In fact, challenge is a sure sign that further development is available. When we relax into the energy of surrender, meaning we release the fight against *what is*, we connect with the power of peace where all things are possible. It is a space where all our channels are open to experience what we require to reach our highest evolution. And my experience has shown me otherworldly protection as I traverse what I need with surrender. I assure you that we will all face unfavorable conditions within our time here on earth, and there is not much we can do to avoid it because all circumstances result from our past actions. In other words, the karma that we have sewn, we shall also reap.

Karma is real, but it's not the bitch it's been made out to be because the results of karma are not just negative. They can also be very positive. Karma is another word to describe the law of cause and effect, and we humans are not exempt from this scientific finding. Every action we take has consequences that return equal reactions. In other words, everything counts. The goal is to accumulate as little karma as possible throughout our life so we can finally rid our souls of the debts we need to pay.

We align with our true nature of goodness when we train our minds through meditation because we connect with the good within us, and this is the nature of the higher mind. We cannot avoid causing harm in this life, just walking on the earth causes harm, but we can lessen it in every area of our life by controlling the mind. Intent affects our energy, and our energy is what the universe is answering at all times.

We are so good at mastering our physical form and know how to use the data and information from our workouts to improve. We know how to periodize training and understand the purposeful flow of building our base to realize a peak of fitness. But what I feel evades most athletes is the true power of controlling the mind and the opportunity we have to be the master of it. Most of us have spent decades in servantry to the mind. We have delighted it with distraction, disappointment, and drama. We have let it breed fear, resistance, and limitation into our reality and given it sovereignty over vital energy that we could otherwise channel toward realizing better performance.

I have seen through my own experience that everything we need to master our minds is already within us. We must go in and retrieve the universal knowledge that resides in our core. We must spend time withdrawing the senses through the stillness of meditation and dedicated mental training. We awaken a part of us that has patiently awaited our attention for decades when we do this. And as we wake up to this dormant Self, we experience qualities of living that are thousands of years ahead of what material science has proven and, at the same time, based on teachings that came thousands of years before material science.

We must give way to the layers we have been clinging to as our worth and realize that they dampen our light and hold us in victimhood. It's the density that must lift and the fog that must clear before we can see. It is a process, often slow, but the air will become clear again if you stay with it. There is no worthy excuse to abandon your pursuit of greatness, and there is no effort that is a waste. There is a perspective that everything is for us, and every day we go to school on this earth to get better. These beliefs are critical to feeling at ease on your journey sooner.

Training as an awake athlete will be the jump you never regret because the sheer velocity of the fall creates resounding changes in the body and mind. Your ability to be your most authentic self will be without effort, and never again will "I'm over it" be a lie that you tell yourself and others. Your "yes" will be "yes," and your "no" will be "no." You will gain trust in the universe and the universe in you. Your word will mean instant manifestation as you realize that your word is your wand, and letting go will be as effortless as blowing dust off a table. You will find a co-creative partnership with the God of your unique understanding as you deepen your relationship with the same energy within you. And as you find a divine organization with your process, you will call your dreams to you at increasing speeds.

You will embody the truth of who you are and burn in the fire of purification more than once along the way. These fires will ask you to let go of your identity as mind and body. And although your willingness to learn will be evident, the ego will fight to the bone for your deepest identifications and worth.

Your narratives and traumas will insist they be energized because a part of you and me believes that it is our wounds that make us special. Rationalizations like this are lies created by the ego, which assumes you need specific markers and characteristics to make you memorable when in truth, you are a reflection of God's light. There is nothing that will make you more special than that. You are uniquely you and loved unconditionally simply because you exist. You will come face to face with the voice of the lower self daily, and it will have you entertaining excuses of why you do not need to meditate. The antidote to this badgering part of us is to become the observer and, as you see with new eyes the terrible master that is the untamed mind, and you will never turn a blind eye to it again.

From the truths you discover, the lies you've been living under will fall away, and it will be easier to set your focus on what you want and not on what you don't want. In time, you will go to your intuition for the answers and gain expertise in sifting and sorting your thought life. Then, just when you think you have it, you will be fooled by your intellect when it demands proof and certainty to measure the results of your efforts. It will discourage you after a messy meditation and tell you that you're not good at it. It would help if you remembered that what you are doing cannot be done by the intellect. The intellect can understand it, which helps to a small degree, but fundamental shifts occur only through experience.

As you take one step at a time, you will better understand the contrast of this physical world and its purpose to help us grow. You will go from being an actor in your life to being the producer of your life experience. Courage and risk will be the not-so-troubling norms of your daily life, and a global pandemic will only confirm your unshakeability. You will no longer choose races through a process of pros and cons because you will understand that the right ones will draw themselves to you based on your point of attraction and the karma you are here to burn. Instead, you will allow your intuition to guide you to your most incredible experience and release the hard lines keeping you small.

Every moment has a purpose, and at some point in your journey, you will be aware that every turn along the way has relevant wisdom to teach. You will be resistant to seeing it sometimes, yet you will get chances time and again to learn what you came here to learn because life unfolds in a way that supports growth. Your higher intelligence will significantly assist you in living beyond unhelpful conditioning and will organize your life experiences to meet such demands. Of course, with every leap of faith, especially this one, there's a massive unknown on the other side, so you should be prepared for moments of immense fear along the way, but over time you will see that those moments teach us how to let go and trust the ride so that it can get better. And you will embrace that uncertainty is the norm living underneath the deluded part of us that desires otherwise.

Because this book is in your hands and you have read this far, I can tell you that you are already the 1% curious about another way to train, race, and live. If you stay open and continue, you may find that you are the 1% of that percent willing to learn how to play this game of life, and perhaps, just perhaps, you'll be the 1% of that percent who becomes the master of their mind—the very one in thousands.

CHAPTER THREE

THE SUPREME SCIENCE

"Yogas citta vritti nirodha: the restraint of the modifications of the mind-stuff is Yoga."

I:2 The Yoga Sutras of Patanjali

Let's talk about science.

The teachings in this book come from my practice of the supreme science, the eight-limbed path of yoga. It is a science of the mind that holds a 5,000-year history in ancient Indian philosophy. Some researchers believe that yoga may be up to 10,000 years old, and others say even more ancient. Yogic teachings are core to my education, which spans over three decades and has transformed me into the person I am today. I am awake. I assure you the veil that kept me in the maya[4] for decades has thinned; through triumph and trauma, I live with a

---

4 Maya, is a spiritual term that can be defined as the dream of being separate; one that denies the interconnectivity of all life. In *The Bhagavad Gita*, as translated by Eknath Easwaran, it is defined as illusion; appearance, as contrasted with reality; the creative power of God.

foot in both worlds—the seen and unseen.

I have come to find my worldly purpose in sharing the teachings of yoga with anyone who is ready and does not mind a direct approach. Beating around the bush has never been my style, and as you dive in with me, you will see that yoga also delivers its wisdom with straight-up simplicity. This chapter's quote is the second sutra, encapsulating yoga's goal; absolute control over the mind which allows us to realize the true Self. The 194 sutras that follow give instructions on how to achieve the goal. Yoga teaches us that we are not the body or the mind but the Seer or the true Self. You, the Seer, are the one that observes your mind and body acting before you, but it does not get involved with what it observes. The Seer is peaceful, and to know yourself as the Seer, your mind must be quiet and clear. It must be devoid of the thought forms that distort the truth of who you are.

To grasp this, Swami Satchidananda asks in the second sutra, "have you ever seen your face?" The answer is no. We have never seen our own face because what we see in the mirror is a reflection. The face is the subject, and the reflection is the object. If the mirror is convex or concave, dirty or broken, we see a distorted reflection of our face. But we do not freak out because we understand it's just the mirror that is distorted, not our face. The same goes for the mind. The Seer is watching the world and experiencing it through the lens of the mind. And so if the mind is mixed up with thoughts and beliefs that distort the truth, who we believe we are will also be distorted. As we practice watching our thoughts, questioning their validity, understanding the ego (I have an entire chapter on that little bugger), and tuning ourselves to quiet through a still practice of meditation, our minds will clear, and we will know our limitless nature beyond doubt.

With yogic science as the base, I pull from discoveries by metaphysicians, quantum physicists, and material scientists to enhance my studies and teaching. Evidence of yoga's benefits and scientific findings keep our intellects engaged, so they are essential. Still, the dedicated practice is what leads us to yoga's enlightening discoveries, and those experiences are beyond the intellect. Yoga accentuates our stamina as athletes because it instructs us not to run away from what feels intense but to stay and relax into those experiences. Whether we do this in motion during a race or in stillness on the cushion, yoga teaches us to watch how we navigate life from the viewpoint of the Seer, without judgment. And we attain this seat of the Self by training our awareness to be on something other than the commentary in our heads, which ultimately yields a quiet, clear mind. It is a masterful finesse, balancing fierce mind control and non-judgment of what we observe.

The very nature of yogic science assists us in seeing what we have not previously seen. These are blind spots in our consciousness. They are misalignments in our physical and mental fitness that keep us from our potential. We so often see this in endurance sports. Unfortunately, athletes are skilled at misaligning with goals. This is because so many of us blindly operate from well-paved neural pathways that keep us in the push-pull struggles of a cluttered, unclear mind. We push when we should rest. We doubt when we know. We pull away when we could be forging ahead at full-speed and fight for our limitations because we are unaware of the lies the ego tells us. Yogic philosophy and the steadfast practice of knowledge in action wake us up to a performance application that rests in the sweet spot between ease and effort, seeking and resisting. In this resting point, we have the clarity to know which choices align with our goals and the strength to choose them.

When I speak about yoga, I am not referring to gymnastics performed in flowy tops with prayer shawls, fabulous jewelry and stretchy pants on earth-friendly rectangles. Despite being a massive fan of all those things, I focus on yoga as a way of living, training, racing, and relating to life in an awakened state. I believe that the body follows the mind; from injury and illness to personal bests and epic feats, what we think becomes our life, inside and out.

I'm not saying that the physical practice of yoga can't change your life. It most certainly does. I was in triangle pose, or trikonasana for you purists, many moons ago in our townhome in Boulder when YogiTriathlete was born. YogiTriathlete is a holistic performance coaching company that is the mothership of Awake Athlete. In a state of present-moment awareness and a pose known as triangle, I realized long-distance triathlon and yoga brought me to the same place from very different directions. An encyclopedia downloaded into my being instantaneously, and without any effort, I accepted a massive shift in the trajectory of my life. I did not know the details. All I knew was that something profound had just occurred.

I was in massage school at BCMT at the time, also working part-time for BJ's web design business, training for triathlons, and recognizing that I was the only triathlete I knew who also practiced yoga. There was undeniable credibility in combining the paths of an athlete with that of a yogi, and I knew it warranted further investigation. The fulfillment of something I felt for a while yet could not articulate was shown to me in that pose in stadium lighting. But it was the mental training of yoga that allowed me to hear my intuition that day and what continues to afford me the courage and patience to follow through to this day. Like all endurance training, mental training is about consistency. Day after day, thought after thought, keep showing up and putting in the time.

Unlike a fartlek[5] workout, the opportunities to apply yogic science to life can be subtle, and if you are not paying close enough attention, you will miss the chance to employ them. Then you will leave a one-star review for this book and slip back into the cyclical patterns that brought you here in the first place. So, let's stay awake, shall we?

Whether you know it or not, we are ever-morphing, ever-expanding organisms en route to a place as familiar as it is foreign. It is a place beyond the conditioning of the human mind and all-encompassing of the universal mind. It is beyond reason, so if we are bound and determined to figure it out first, we will forever be stuck in the mind.

---

5 Fartlek means "speed-play" in Swedish. It is a style of endurance run training where specific intervals of faster speeds are mixed in with intervals of slower speeds. The purpose behind this type of training is to condition the body to run faster speeds over longer distances.

I used to believe that physical activity ushered in mental training. So when I stepped up mentally in a workout or a race, I thought that was mental training when really I was just enduring the unpleasant and waiting impatiently for something to change. It had nothing to do with being masterful about my relationship to pain, embodying that I am not the body, or being in a non-judgemental state of mind. At the time, I did not see mind training as foundational or as a unique discipline, even though I had practiced yoga since the early 1990s. I was staying on the surface with my mental game. I was tough, no doubt, and described as an optimist, but I was nowhere near being the master of my mind.

As we train the mind and attune to a quieter environment through meditation, the ultra-fine voice of the Seer gains more presence in our life. Yoga instructs that we find this voice in the stillness, and if we spend enough time there, we will hear it everywhere. And although I am describing it as a voice, it's more of a state of knowing. Stay with the practice, and you'll see what I'm talking about in time. Many of us live with the awareness of our intuitive voice now, but we are not acting on it. We do not act on the intuitive voice or gut feelings because we do not trust them, and this is because we do not trust ourselves. And this all makes sense, right? I mean, how can we trust ourselves when we have not discovered or embraced all of who we are? And if we do not fully know who we are, how can we truly know anything?

The awakening you are moving into is a new way of living and viewing the world with an underlying curiosity for truth. It is a grand recognition that we have a say in how we experience our lives and that we can consciously align our actions toward what we desire. When we do this from a connected relationship with Self, we align with our soul's purpose or dharma, and from there, we unearth the gifts we came here to share.

This can seem like a lot, and I have talked to many who carry pressure to find their purpose or feel lost because they have not yet discovered it, but you guys, it's okay. We never were taught how to connect with our intuitive awareness. Instead, we learned that knowledge was outside of us, and we had to put it in so we could be smart and successful in the world. So it feels risky when we act on our intuition, especially when we are just starting and always when it does not add up on paper. This is where the guidance of a teacher also walking the path is helpful and necessary.

Intuition is learning from within; it is subtle. It has nothing to do with what you have and is far superior to societal ideals. We are programmed to look outside ourselves for satisfaction and happiness. Yoga teaches us the opposite; it directs us within and reminds us that the world outside merely reflects our world inside.

I hope you will attend many yoga classes in the future to put the themes in this book into practice. Yoga studios are inherently safe, and our nervous systems feel that safety. As we feel safe, we feel calm, and in the quiet of calmness, we receive the benefits of yoga, not the least of which occurs on a cellular level. It is true; science has revealed that yoga positively and significantly impacts our cellular health. One example is how meditation and mindful practices reduce stress and therefore assist in healing stress-related cellular damage in our bodies. To prove this concept, engage with the tools in this book and experience the mind-body shifts from your awakened responses to life's stressors. Another way is a simple search on the internet. Here you will find many scientific conclusions that confirm the same. But as Hindu sage, Ramana Maharshi, reminded us in the quote I used for the introduction of this book, we will not realize of our true Self from reading about it. It's not in a book, it is through experience that we awaken.

The term yoga means to yoke or bring together for a means of a purpose. In our case, as awake athletes, it means to direct more focus towards awareness of our subtle Self and away from focusing on our ego and human self as our whole. From this we gain conscious access to our boundless nature as the means to navigate the circumstances of life.

It's not a renunciation of society and worldly possessions, nothing that extreme. Yoga simply provides us with a set of guidelines and practices for living that puts the mind into the role of servantry where it is supposed to be so that we can realize the truth of who we are: limitless, all-knowing, and ever-powerful. Yoga is not hocus pocus or a religion or anything that requires robes and a cave. It is a sophisticated science of the mind comprised of the following eight limbs:

1) Yama - right living

2) Niyama - positive duties

3) Asana - posture practice

4) Pranayama - breath control

5) Pratyahara - sense withdrawal

6) Dharana - concentration

7) Dhyana - meditation

8) Samadhi - contemplation

The first two limbs, the yamas, and niyamas, are ten elementary instructions for life. When I first heard of these guidelines, I thought of the Ten Commandments and the Bible, which did not sit well with me as the Christian commandments were a source of fear for me growing up. I was told to memorize them, which I did, but in my imperfection as a human, I saw that I had already violated some of them. I had senselessly killed mosquitoes and spiders; I didn't realize they were souls on a journey just like me. I had definitely not honored my mother and father because I didn't always do what they told me, and sometimes I got mad at them. I had taken the lord's name in vain and heard it taken that way often in my home, and Sundays never felt holy to me, so I must have been doing something wrong. And what about the other days of the week? Were they less than Sunday? I felt disconnected from something the church told me was the most important connection. I internalized my violations and decided I must be a bad person (kid), so I hid them. In anticipation of impending doom on Judgment Day, I developed a deep fear and resentment toward them.

Thankfully, MB assured me that yoga is not an organized religion, which was a great relief because when we started working with each other in my late 30s, I was still so confused about my Catholic upbringing. He assured me these ten tenets were beautiful guides for living a powerful life aligned with universal law. He also helped me understand that the Ten Commandments are not scary; my misled belief about them fueled my fear. He met my concerns and fears without judgment, and the knowledge he imparted to me during our sessions helped me to understand that no one was sending me to walk the plank anytime soon. As I learned more about these tenets, I saw a pathway for me to live freely, and I hope these ten assist you in finding the same.

The first of these gems is the five yamas which guide us to move through the world aligned with our true nature. They are practices that shine a light on whether we are making a negative impact on the world or a positive impact.

1) Ahimsa - non-violence

2) Satya - non-lying

3) Asteya - non-stealing

4) Brahmacharya - non-excess

5) Aparigraha - non-possessiveness

The second of these sacred tenets is the niyamas which are the observances. They teach us to turn inward and open to fine-tuning ourselves through cognizance of our inner reality.

1) Saucha - purity

2) Santosha - contentment

3) Tapas - self-discipline

4) Svadhyaya - self-study

5) Ishvara Pranidhana - surrender

The yamas and niyamas are ripe for embodiment in all we do, including training and racing. They are escorts to move in a specific direction in life; mastery. They keep us on point with being our best, and I promise they will make you strong. They guide us in being connected human beings who are awake to the lives and well-being of others as well as the voice of the deluded mind. The deluded mind is the voice of the small self. It is the voice of the ego and I will expand more later. The thing to know now is that the ego is not your enemy, and it can be your teammate if you tame it.

Together the yamas and the niyamas set the stage for serenity as each offers balance to our experience. The energy of each is pure and clean. When put into action, these tenets are a pro-health way to live. Increased health means less time spent in injury and illness, which means more time training and racing. For an in-depth and commonsensical understanding of these ten guidelines, check out *The Yamas And Niyamas* by Deborah Adele, which is on the booklist at the end of this book.

The third limb of yoga is asana, or the physical postures of yoga. Whatever gets you to the mat is good; beer yoga, hot yoga, yin yoga, cross-training, injury, sadness, etc. It doesn't matter what guides you to an asana practice; if you stick with it, you will see that the poses are just the vehicle for the practice. And over time, this understanding will naturally follow you off the mat and into the poses of your life.

The modern-day yoga experience of moving from pose to pose is not as ancient as you may think and perhaps completely different from the true meaning of asana. In spiritual texts and scripture like the *Bhagavad Gita, Upanishads*, and *The Yoga Sutras of Patanjali*, the only reference to asana is a sitting posture for meditation, a relaxed yet activated posture taken solely to reach higher states of consciousness by making the mind one-pointed. The postures most commonly seen in formal practice came from a few movements in the late 19th and early 20th centuries. Namely, gymnastic conditioning from the Brits and the Danes, ancient Indian traditions combined with physical activities like wrestling, and a 20th-century belief that building stronger bodies would make for a stronger nation. These, along with influencers on western culture like T. Krishnamacharya, who is said to be the first to pair movement with breath in a yoga class, and his students, namely B.K.S. Iyengar and Pattabhi Jois, all came together to create the physical practice so often seen today. Whether you are active on a mat or still in meditation, asana disciplines the mind, it brings awareness into our bodies as a reminder that we are living through a body and teaches us to remain calm in the face of sensation, a particularly potent skill for athletes.

The fourth limb of yoga is pranayama. *Prana* is our life energy or life force, the breath of life, and *yama* pertains to the "practice of." Pranayama aids the management of life energy by controlling the rhythms of breath through different exercises. As we put our focus and will on the breath, just like anything, we will learn more about it. As we learn about the breath, we deepen our experience with life force that feeds the breath and is the unchanging energy of our true Self.

Additionally, breath is an anchor to the present moment because breath is always happening right now. If we put 100% of our awareness on the breath, we will be 100% present. When fully present, we can experience life independently of the commentary in our heads. When we operate independently of the commentary, our thoughts no longer dictate our actions without our conscious permission. Therefore, it is safe to say that if we control the breath, we can control our thoughts; when we control our thoughts, we control the mind, thus the goal of yoga.

Furthermore, operating independently of the thinking mind means we have created a gap between the commentary and our awareness. It amplifies our influence over the voice of the conditioned mind and allows us to concentrate our focus where we want it and when we want it there. This leads to increased flow experiences where activity and awareness merge and optimal performance transpires.

The fifth limb of yoga is pratyahara. This one can take a minute to digest. For me, it's taken years. It means withdrawing the senses from objects by directing our senses inward instead of outward into the physical world. Earth, this physical realm, is a three-dimensional world and we live it through our human body, which lives through the senses. We smell an Italian restaurant nearby, and we crave garlic bread. We see the latest and greatest running shoes, and we must have them. We feel the fabric of our new triathlon kit and cannot wait to put it on. We hear our teammates talk about their latest trail race, and we instantly sign up for the following year. We taste the salty chips at an aid station and can't wait to get to the next one, so we can have more.

Living through the senses taps into our animal instinct, leaving us in a constant state of desire. It feels carnal, and I have come to know that it is just one aspect of me. I never thought of it that way until I began to get to know the other part of myself, which is the opposite of carnal. It is non-aggressive, patient as all get out, and yet somehow more powerful than anything I've touched before. And it is in me. And it is in you. It is the part that lives beneath the senses because it created the senses and is the living force behind them.

The desire for more is not necessarily negative as it aids our athletic endeavors and, most definitely, the path of awakening.

Once I told my teacher I was taking my daily 45-minute meditation to a 60-minute practice, he immediately said, "no." He explained that we want to preserve the longing because it will drive us to continue. And so, waking up is not about kicking the human part of us to the curb; it is about utilizing our human design to our advantage. We will always want more, and this is not to say that we cannot celebrate the day our new bike arrives or the moment when we step off the plane into a tropical race destination; by all means, enjoy the luxuries of life. We live in an ever-changing world; please indulge in the physical fruits of manifestation, but know that you do not have to respond to every impulse along the way. Pratyahara is a profound slowing down and drawing attention inward; it is here we find spaciousness. This connection helps us to get into the gap between stimulus and response.

The week of taper[6] leading into a race is one of my favorite times to practice this limb. I keep my power under control through pratyahara by building energy without releasing my inner animal too soon. I withdraw my senses from social media chatter. I notice but do not indulge in the cravings I experience to expend unnecessary energy or eat foods that will not serve my race day performance. Instead, I meditate more and turn my focus inward to stoke my fire.

I feel sensation build inside me that peaks to a point where I think I may explode, and I practice pranayama to expand calmness. In that calmness, I have tremendous power to

6 Taper is a phase in endurance training when, the days leading into a competition, exercise is reduced to allow the athlete the restoration needed for optimal performance.

self-regulate. The stimulus builds, and I practice not
responding. It builds more, and I practice not responding. I do
what coaches instruct their athletes to do, I save it for race day,
and pratyahara helps me do that better than ever.

When I think of pratyahara, I often think of the movie
Braveheart, specifically, the battle scene when Mel Gibson
holds his army back as their opponent races toward them at
increasing speeds. Mel's army obeys the command; they remain
still yet visibly on edge. He repeats the order, "hold," four times.
Then, at the very last moment, he unleashes the battle cry. Mel
and his army kneel, pick up their spears, and the enemy runs
directly into them, meeting their demise. In this example, Mel
is your higher Self, powerfully commanding you to chill out and
trust that the right action will occur at the exact right moment.
The enemy is your untamed animal within, and I have learned
that it is best to get our inner animal tame to our command if
we desire top performance in our sport and life because to be
masterful, we must be the master of our mental faculties.

The sixth limb of yoga is dharana or concentration. This
limb is essential for athletes and ties very well into pratyahara.
Remain focused on the big goal without indulging the
distractions that vie for your attention. With this limb, we
make great strides in taming the ego and shining a light on the
conditioning that no longer serves our dreams.

The goal of yoga is to cease the mental fluctuations, still the
mind, and concentrate within the silence of any life experience.
It is a practice that evolves over a long time, so please, relax. It

will take a minute to calm the unhelpful momentum previously created by your ego. The mind is a tricky bugger deeply conditioned to be distracted and entertained. So when you remove stimuli, you can expect a fight, but patience will assist you in attaining the goal of complete mind control.

When the mind is untrained, it is busy with thoughts. It is like a monkey swinging in the jungle from branch to branch. It flies through the air, grasping onto whatever vine is in its close vision—a new bike, carbon-plated shoes, your competition, latest age group rankings, course changes, race day unknowns—any of these are possibilities for the monkey. It does not care; as long as it clings to something, it will feel safe for a while. It will feel peace until another desire arises, the fear of missing out takes over, or comparison energy pins you as *more than* or *less than*, and then the ripples will rise again. When we consider the ceasing of fluctuations or modifications of the mind-stuff, I imagine a still pond, as clear and smooth as glass. Now, imagine a fish jumping up through the water's surface, making a big splash. Ripples disrupt the pristine nature of the pond, but the pond doesn't complain, doesn't cry victim, and doesn't get anxious. The pond allows the ripples to be there until they are not, at which time it returns to its clear and undisturbed nature.

The difference between the pond and our minds is that left to its own devices, the mind will live through the senses influenced by external circumstances and identify with mental preferences. It will relate to the ego as itself, the distorted reflection of our nature, and therefore, it will swing into the fray from vine to vine with attention scattered and absence of focus.

Patanjali, Indian sage and father of modern yoga, describes the monkey mind as the mental modifications, or the vritti, that get in the way of our ability to concentrate and, ultimately, our ability to raise our consciousness and accept the world as it is without judgment. Vritti is Sanskrit for whirlpool, and this is what we so often experience when we sit for meditation. We get still with the best intentions, and then the whirlpool of mental fluctuations captures our focus. And so, as we catch ourselves caught up in the swirling and swinging nature of the monkey mind, we concentrate again. And again. Over time we will develop excellent skills within this limb of the practice, which is necessary for our success as athletes. Think about it, if we cannot focus our mind when doing nothing, how do we expect to purposefully concentrate on what we want during the swim of a triathlon or at mile 35 of a 100k endurance run?

When we practice dharana, we place our mental monkey on a vine and keep it there while not allowing any thought to penetrate our focus. I often remind my mind when practicing dharana that there is no thought more important than what I am doing, absolutely no thought more important. This takes a strong dose of self-will, but you already possess this as a natural strength; otherwise, you would not be reading this book open to training the mind like the 1%.

The practice of concentration is the precursor to the quiet of meditation or, as quantum physics refers to it, zero-state awareness. This silent expanse is tricky because the moment we realize we are in the state of meditation, a state of no mind, we are no longer in that state. This goes the same for athletic flow states; when we realize we are in flow, we are no longer in flow. Flow, like meditation, is a state where the mind is one-pointed. So it is when activity and awareness merge, without any focus on thoughts. Our energy and faculties are entirely concentrated on the experience of the moment, which creates a state devoid of physical, mental, and emotional restrictions.

We practice concentration on the meditation cushion, but we can also practice it in our training. Yes, we can increase our rate of flow in life and sport. In running, for example, it is the practice of holding a one-pointed focus (awareness) on each foot strike (activity). This takes practice, but the best way to get better at deliberately focusing your awareness is to begin. So, during your next training session, and let's stay with the running example, put 100% of your awareness on your foot strike and return your full attention to it each time you find yourself drifting into thought. Rinse and repeat.

Without training the mind to concentrate, states of meditation and flow will be few and far between. And so, what most people do when they meditate is primarily the practice of concentration—focusing the mind on breath, mantra, the flame of a candle, etc. These are all practices of concentration. Only when the mind is calm enough will it slip into the state of meditation, which takes us to our next limb.

The seventh limb of yoga is meditation, a practice that I wholeheartedly believe is the most critical thing we can do as humans to better the whole. It is the basis of the work in this book and an accelerator to decelerating the pace of the monkey mind. I have not found a substitute for sitting in stillness every day. Meditation is calming for our mind, body, and spirit. Calm is the frequency of our all-knowing, intuitive Self or Seer. As we spend more time in stillness and silence, our intuition becomes the primary voice that directs our training, racing, and life while the monkey follows our command. We move from being an actor in our life to the producer of our life experience.

Meditation connects us to something greater than our human beingness. It puts us into concert with our eternal nature that resides beneath and within the depths of everything we know and believe about being human. In stillness, we accustom ourselves to our essence which cannot be felt in a *go, go, go* life. It is an all-knowing force that does not beg for our attention but patiently awaits our attention. It is the energy of our source. It is the energy of all that is, ever was, and ever will be. It is the only still point within an ever-moving, ever-changing world. The practice of meditation takes us to stillness through stillness. It brings us home from where we came and allows us to exist in authenticity and genuine truth.

The eighth and final limb of yoga is samadhi, or the joyful state of yoga. It is the precursor to self-realization when one's potential is fulfilled. It comes in several stages following deep forms of meditation. It is evident in the body through the ceasing of breath when all layers of delusion fall away, and we sustain in this physical world through prana or life force alone.

As a result of the disciplined practices of yoga, we purify the mind and body. As we do this, our physical cells absorb more life force, our consciousness rises, and our vibration elevates. Our ability to experience the world and all we encounter without judgment free us from the shackles of the mind.

Equal application of all yogic limbs is recommended because they work off one another as a complete recipe for the mastery of life. Yoga is the map, and we are the travelers. The map's legend is living through the guides of the yamas and niyamas, strengthening physical discipline through asana, managing life force through breath, directing the senses inward with pratyahara, making the mind one-pointed through dhrana, experience meditative states, and then access contemplative samadhi. Follow this map steadfastly, and the fluctuations of your mind-stuff will cease, and liberation from all that holds you back as an athlete and human will abide.

Every step and stage along the way is progress, and I encourage you to use everything to your advantage. Each training session, competition, life challenge, and success is here for you to grow and expand. Live in constant wonder and curiosity about who you are, and never stop aspiring to realize your absolute potential.

We are all here on purpose and for a purpose; that purpose is our dharma. The yogis believe that everyone has unique dharma and that it is better to fail at being you than succeed in trying to live the path of another. We are here to fulfill our dharma and pay our karmic debts while not accumulating more. I recognize how challenging it is not to get caught up in the drama of life's circumstances. There is a part of each of us that finds it all so delicious, I know, but this is what keeps us identified with the fluctuating mind.

Swami Satchidananda said that all yoga practices are to maintain a tranquil mind in all situations. It is in this calmness that we tap into the Self. The one that observes all and exists within the remembrance that we are powerful beings meant to co-create our lives alongside the universe by being the masters of our minds.

I have yet to work with an athlete who does not desire more calm in their life. We all seek it, but most seek it in the wrong places. We seek it through accomplishment, material things, and approval, none of which bring sustainable peace. The only peace with staying power is the peace within, and the only true freedom is the freedom from our minds. It is the freedom that we all seek, and yoga, the supreme science of the mind, shows us the way.

CHAPTER FOUR

A NEW WORLDVIEW

"Nothing stands between man and his highest ideals and every desire of his heart, but doubt and fear. When man can wish without worrying, every desire will be instantly fulfilled."

Florence Scovel Shinn

To be faster, more competitive, confident, calm, whatever it may be that we desire, we must first decide that we can have it. Once that is accomplished, we must remain steadfast in our focus to have it. If we scatter our focus by rethinking our desires, doubting our ability to attain them, or worse, giving up on our dreams, our results will also be scattered. Dharana plays a vital role in our ability to reach our goals because increasing concentration equals less distraction, which is the most streamlined way to manifest our desires.

An essential piece of manifesting is to know the mechanics needed to bring a desire into reality are born as soon as the desire is born. And if you can stay focused and nullify doubt, trusting the process will become second nature. Look, I know it can be scary, and I know that sometimes what life calls us to seems unreasonable. Painful even. I mean, have you ever run an ultra marathon? Started a blog? Shared a secret? Risked stability for a dream? I have, and I understand what it feels like to have no idea where to start, but that doesn't warrant quitting before you start. Instead, move forward despite all the excuses not to begin, and if you don't know where to start, then start by feeling what you desire.

To be a better runner, we must practice feeling into the persona of a better runner. We have to adopt an abundance mindset to have an abundant bank account. To get to the starting line of the Ultra Trail du Mont Blanc (UTMB) endurance run, we must become a UTMB competitor in our words, thoughts, actions, and feelings. Take time in your meditation practice once or twice weekly to envision what you desire and practice feeling that vision as if you are already living it. Then take those feelings into your every day as you also logically work towards your goals through action.

For the awake athlete who desires to be a better runner, you can practice feeling the fluidity in your body that you see in the body of your favorite runner. Ask yourself, how does that runner dress for their runs, and how do they feel in those clothes? How do they feel as they slide their feet into their shoes and take their first few strides? You must recruit your imagination to practice this identity creation, and if you do, you become that runner today in feeling. If you stay with it, the physical evidence will catch up to the feeling of your vibration and then shine through in your performance.

For those who no longer desire to live in financial lack and worry, ask yourself if you are willing to imagine and feel a life where financial stress does not exist. And then, feel that life. Take time to tune yourself to abundance. Observe the blades of grass in a park, leaves on a tree, drops of water in the ocean, and sand in the desert. Feel the limitless abundance of this natural world and know that you are not separate from that abundance. Take action in the physical world, become the CEO of your bank account and open your eyes and mind to embody the truth of what is. There is no lack in this universe, only in our minds.

For the runner that desires to line up at UTMB, imagine and feel the crisp air of the French Alps. How does it feel when it hits your teeth? Can you hear the other runners breathing around you as you endeavor an ascent? How does it feel to stop at your first breathtaking view and absorb the majesty of the mountains? Can you feel your trekking poles secured to your hands and the powerful energy of the supporters? You do not have to wait for the physical reality to arrive; you can be there now.

If our dreams are always in the future, the future is where they will stay. Envisioning, instead of just visioning, is the addition of tuning our frequency to match the frequency of what it is we desire. We do this through feeling and then back it up with our words, actions, and thoughts. This process invites our dreams to run toward us instead of us always having to chase them down.

And as we embody what we desire as if we already possess it, the space we previously reserved for doubt and negative thought narrows considerably because when we stop focusing on what we do not want, we start attracting what we do want.

Life and how we live it are akin to the sport of Boomerang; what we throw out into the world through our thoughts, words, and actions is what we receive in return. Yoga calls it karma or the law of cause and effect. The Bible describes it as "whatsoever a man soweth, that shall he also reap." In quantum physics, it's the law of attraction; in material science, it's Newton's Third Law; there is an equal and opposite reaction for every action.

Albert Einstein, one of the greatest physicists who ever lived, proclaimed that everything is energy. Therefore, to attain what we desire, all we have to do is match its frequency, and it will manifest into our reality. He went on to say that this was not philosophy but physics. And we have made it commonplace to exist in denial of this fundamental law. We live life like we are guaranteed a tomorrow and run our mouths without regard for the power of our words. We doubt our dreams and those of others without recognizing that our essence is creative energy; therefore, we create in each moment.

Our words, actions, and thoughts are the precursors to what comes next. There is no overriding law, but there is a way to work alongside physical and metaphysical laws. There is a mindset that does not wait for the other shoe to drop, one that knows we are here to discover our power to create and our birthright to manifest. A perspective that sees the only limits that exist are the limits in our minds. It is a view of our life's journey that understands any dream that sits within our hearts is there for a reason. And each moment, we either move closer or further away from its expression.

It is a new worldview that may be new to you, and it is a mindset that leads to a *both/and* reality. It is a way of being that does not sit around and wait for something to happen, nor does it play victim to the belief that it's only up to us to realize our dreams. It adheres to other metaphysical laws like the law of least effort, which teaches us the recipe for manifestation; ask, allow, receive. As I mentioned before, that factor of karma comes into play, so if your dream doesn't come to fruition right away or it feels like you are derailed along the way, stay with it; you are simply off-gassing the results of past actions. As Einstein taught, if you keep steady with your vision, it will manifest into your reality.

There are many markers along the way to gauge where you are with a manifestation. By watching your words, paying attention to your responses, and feeling your actions, you will see just how far on or off par you are with your dreams because you will see if you are flowing with or pushing against the cosmic stream from which all manifests. With an observant eye on life, I promise you the clarity of your path will come naturally. Patterns and life circumstances will begin to make more sense as the evidence of all you have created thus far is revealed. It is pretty simple, but this simplicity becomes an impossibility when we identify with the conditioned mind, which is built on a foundation of limitation.

If we train our minds to stay out of the realms of doubt and negative thought by redirecting the mind when we find it dwelling in the realms of doubt and negative thought, we can have whatever we desire. We must believe it to see it. To do this, we recruit and use our faculty of imagination, which draws the reality to us. Athletes have been doing this for decades. Visionaries, for centuries. To see it beforehand is the essence of visualization. Going through an event in our mind's eye, rehearsing our race, and responding calmly to the obstacles that may come our way are effective techniques to train the mind and prime the body.

Visualization can decrease pre-race anxiety while boosting confidence and enhancing motivation to achieve what you want. As far as your brain is concerned, visualizing is the same as the actual event. Your body uses the same neurons when you imagine your desires as when they play out in reality. Add the practice of feeling your dreams as part of your reality now instead of believing that they are in the future, and you will tune your frequency and attain what you desire faster than ever before.

For the science buffs, remember, this is not philosophy; this is physics, but it is not how the masses manifest. Most people choose an old worldview where they create their lives by default through old ways of thinking and relying on programs that no longer align with who they are or where they desire to be in life. They cling to the vision of the small self by associating with conditioning from their past and denying there is a bigger plan at play.

To hold a new worldview is to live awake to our co-creative partnership with the universe. It is the unrelenting quest to know and live in truth as we see it in each moment. It is an ever-morphing path that forever unfolds the layers of delusion that cloud our relationship with source energy as our creator and co-pilot. It is a movement towards a greater understanding that everything is for us. It means we stop resisting hardship and clinging to joy. Instead, we embody that there are only lessons to garner from this life and that we can train our minds to welcome all things. My yoga mentor, Philip, teaches this very thing; he says the highest state of spiritual intelligence is to welcome all things. This resonated when I heard it because I realized I did not want to endure life anymore or just make do; I wanted to welcome. I wanted to reach the highest state. Something about it felt easeful and spacious, like I could breathe better. And now I do.

Through the years, I learned that we are individualized reflections of source light and are loved unconditionally simply because we exist. Unfortunately, this eternal truth is forgotten by most, doubted by the rest, and often lost in defensive confusion around the rules of religion. Being an awake athlete has nothing to do with religion, except if you listen closely, you will hear that we all deliver the same message; all things are possible when we are in concert with our highest intelligence which is always in a welcoming state.

To truly awaken to a new worldview, we must know the old worldview, the one soaking in the marinade of *either/or*. A limited view that says you can't have your cake and eat it too. It says rich people are jerks, and top-level athletes must be selfish. It is an excuse-a-tarian addict because it does not believe life can be that good. It is full of effort, and rarely is anything good enough. It is disappointed with finish times, attached to expectations, and completely disregards that the present moment is anything more than a time frame to rehash the past or rehearse the future. It falls scared in the face of success and declares that we must see it first to believe it.

The old worldview is the new world's shadow and guides its adopters along the heavy path, the one that makes sense on paper. Rarely does it throw caution to the wind and risk everything to go after its dreams. This is the passage of the masses. Nevertheless, it manages to accomplish a lot considering its exhausting nature, but I would be remiss not to share with you that it is not the only way to live and create.

We all incarnated into a world of contrast: love and hate, darkness and lightness, beauty and ugliness, horror and delight. There is no question that there is hell on this earth. For some, hell manifests in their physical environments, but for many, it is the incessant neural looping of negative old world thoughts that create patterns of dissatisfaction in their lives. To be free of the self-induced push-pull struggles of the mind, we must decide to live from the 10,000-foot perspective so we can see more of the story as it unfolds for us.

The new worldview supports us in doing what we love because it says we unearth our gifts when we find ease and joy, no matter what we must traverse in the unearthing process. As we unearth our gifts, we open to purpose. Our gifts come in infinite ways. It's up to us to go in, find them, and share them bravely. Take action, and the universe will conspire to support you. The awake athlete path, which sees with a new worldview, asks us to become an archeologist of Self. A little bit every day, over a long period of time, we chip away. We feel what lies within our hearts; if we listen closely, we will hear the subtle energy of limitlessness guiding us at every step. If we apply what we find to our athletic performance, we enter the realm of our potential. Even though some of your dreams and future endeavors may feel entirely out of reach today, rest assured that you will excavate limitations and become open to possibilities through self-study. We have permission from the universe to live the life of our dreams, and it helps those who help themselves. It assists us after we make the first move. And in my experience, that first move always involves direction from my heart and risk because it rarely is the plan that makes sense on paper.

For example, I held a knowing for decades that I would live in California at some point. I kept this knowledge to myself for most of those years, only sharing it once or twice. Because, have you noticed? Many people have many opinions about California. At least that's what I noticed growing up in New England, and most of those did not help me realize my dream, so I kept quiet about it. I had no concrete plan of when or how; I just knew that when it was time, I would know, just like how I knew when the opportunity to go to India presented itself.

In the meantime, even before I knew anything about
universal law or meditation, I noticed unhelpful thoughts and
conditioned beliefs I had about California and practiced new
thoughts that were helpful. I counteracted "California is too
expensive" with "millions of people live in California, and
so can I." And "California has earthquakes" with "I grew up
with annual hurricanes, and not only survived those hurricanes
but celebrated those times of hunkering down." And just as I
suspected for many years, it came with clarity when the time
arrived to take the leap.

It was December of 2015, and BJ and I had just returned
from racing IRONMAN⁷ Cozumel for our 13th wedding
anniversary, a trip preceded by letting go of our dear Bernese
Mountain dog, Lhasa. I was five years into my meditation
journey, two years into my career as a yoga teacher, and steadily
winding down my massage therapy practice. My yoga following
grew, and I was paid well for my classes. I developed a popular
"Yoga for Athletes" workshop; our status as vegan athletes was
gaining more attention in the community, and YogiTriathlete
was on the cusp of becoming a company. Until then, it was my
blog where I wrote about the intersection between endurance
sports and yoga. Yet during this time of professional success
and financial freedom, I could not help but feel I had hit a
spiritual ceiling that I was banging into daily. Something inside
me was yearning for a grand adventure and massive risk, but
I had no idea what that was, and I was starting to feel lost and
alone.

---

7 IRONMAN is a brand name of triathlon, in the case of the IRONMAN races named in this
book it refers to the triathlon comprised of a 2.4 mile swim, 112 mile bike and a 26.2 mile run.

BJ was working a corporate job with a comforting salary and incredible benefits. He was slightly shy of becoming 100% vested in the company through its employee stock ownership plan, which meant considerable dollars were lurking around the corner. On paper, BJ should still be there, reaping the financial and professional rewards of a wonderful company whose leaders respected him greatly, but the truth was, his heart was longing to pursue a dream to be a coach. He was finding disharmony in a situation that society told him should not be abandoned. But, as we soon discovered, the universe had different plans than what society deemed safe and sound. A cosmic inspiration that supported his dream to leap and freed me from the ceiling that blocked my expansion. It appeared to me on a wintery New England afternoon just days after returning from Cozumel, amid deep meditation, I saw the word "California." I can still remember the font lit by the brightest of light. I stayed for the remainder of the time because I felt a peace I was not ready to wake from, but when I did, I picked up my phone and texted BJ.

My message read, "I got a plan. We're outta here."

Immediately, three dancing dots appeared.

He replied, "I'm in as long as it's warm."

When he came home that night, he asked me about the plan. I shared the vision I received but told him there were few details of how it was to unfold. I felt confident that more information was forthcoming. I just needed to continue to sit every day.

The details came within the week but differed from what the logical mind would expect. There was no concrete plan, only an undeniable ask from a higher force to serve others as we lept into our dream. It was a dream we could only feel then; it was nothing we could articulate. We knew everything was changing, and something profound was en route, so trust was the only option. It was bigger than us, and it certainly was not as clean as one would hope, like selling our home and getting on a plane to the west coast with money in the bank. Instead, it became a cross-country adventure about raising awareness that living a more vibrant life is within reach for all. And the trip itself became known as the Ride The High Vibe Tour.

On June 14, 2016, we loaded our Honda Fit with everything we owned—two carry-on suitcases, Clark and his backpack, our triathlon race bags, race bikes on the roof, camping equipment, podcast gear, our Vitamix, a handful of books, a Tibetan singing bowl from my trip to India, a small statue of the Buddha, incense, sage and a boat load of faith. We closed on the sale of our home that morning, and I think it's essential to add that this house was my dream home. A home I never thought I would leave. But alas, we sold the house, quit our jobs, left our families and friends, rid ourselves of most of our material possessions, except what we fit in our Fit, and hit the road.

No digital pictures of pictures. No love letters from our dating years. No storage unit. No plan, no budget, and no timeline. But we had each other and a commitment to keep all channels open and say "yes" to the flow of life. There was something inescapably exciting about putting ourselves in this position. BJ and I both knew if we stayed awake to the miracle of each day, we'd realize a life we never thought possible. And in case you are wondering, we have discovered that life. I assure you, it was not without challenge but with unwavering faith and belief in the possibilities of the unknown, we received blessings every day, and they started even before we departed.

During the last class I taught at Rhode Island Power Yoga, the students presented us with a hefty jar of money for gas and an unlimited supply of encouragement for our venture. When we arrived in Lake Placid, NY, our first stop, we came to know the local bike shop owners who happened to have a yoga studio on the second floor and were looking to offer more classes. We put up flyers around town, I offered a mindfulness workshop, and I was honored to guide locals, tourists, and young athletes from Quebec during their summer training camp.

The word spread as we continued to make our way across the country, whipping up green smoothies in the bathrooms of campgrounds and inspiring people to minimize excess for more breathing room in their environment. Vibrancy was revealing itself in so many ways. People reached out and asked if they could send us money to support our mission. We had a family in Utah open up their 12,000-square-foot mansion to us for as long as we'd like, and the mother didn't really like dogs. But if you know Clark, you know he's a natural charmer. We had another couple in Ventura, CA, the brother of one of my Rhode Island students, move out for Thanksgiving and give us their home for the holiday. These wonderful people also introduced us to the coffee game-changer known as Chemex. We did not know where to sleep many nights, and then a hotel would appear at the perfect price.

Throughout it all, we were willing to be taken off course and serve wherever we felt a pull, but thankfully that pull guided us to Carlsbad, California, a town we had never heard of before arriving in San Diego. There are so many stories surrounding this six-month adventure that we could not have scripted. We bravely embraced the new world mindset without compromise. As a result, we welcomed incredible miracles and proved what we had heard from others living their dream; when you follow a deep calling from within, the universe will conspire to support you.

We had no plan B; it was YogiTriathlete all the way, and that came with significant challenges in the financial department. But as we continued to focus on what we wanted, which pulled our focus away from what we didn't want, we were awake to receive blessings as they poured in. I remember one day receiving a check in the mail for over a thousand dollars from an overpayment on our Rhode Island homeowners insurance which I used to pay our rent for the month. Our willingness to stay the course, believe in the stream of well-being and embody that there is no lack in this universe blessed us greatly. As a result, we became stewards of a brand, now plural with the birth of Awake Athlete, that assists those ready to shift their mindsets from limitation to limitlessness. From an old to a new worldview.

The new world mind embraces that a co-creative partnership means a two-way street. It knows that so much is streaming towards you now: your dreams, fears, and doubts. Through joy and challenge, life will call us all to more, but when we embrace that everything is energy, and although we cannot create or destroy energy, we also embrace that we can transform it. And as we transform the energy of our thoughts and train our minds through mindful practices and expanded perspectives, we transform our energetic resonance to a higher vibration, and thus our stream becomes cleaner. This is the stage in life when you hear people tell you, "I love your energy" or "I want your life." At this point, you will naturally inform everyone you meet that they can live the life they want, just like you. And that it can start right now. We cannot force anyone to adopt an awake mindset, but for those who are ready, we get to see the shift from the old to the new world right before our eyes. And despite the obstacles along the way, there will be ease because they realize, like I have, that living with anything but a new world mind is suffering.

This brave new world welcomes infinite success and joy into our lives without compromise. And even though you may think you are doing that now, I promise you that if you are not meditating and deepening your relationship with the present moment, you are not seeing the compromises you are making all over the place. A new worldview adopts the perspective of all perspectives because it is the state of an expanded being, and expansion is a process achieved only through experience.

To live connected to infinite possibility, you must understand

that you will be living against the grain. Not everyone will
get you; people will fall away from your life as they argue for
their *either/or* old world beliefs. Set the intent to be okay with
whatever happens along this path and trust that your power
is in your ability to choose your response to life. A new world
mind calls for us to release all feelings of victimhood because
only then can we tune ourselves to the frequency of universal
power where no victim exists. We all have equal power within.
The light of our source is shining on all of us the same.

When we live from a new world perspective, we understand
that we are powerful, energetic beings. We take full ownership
that our past responses to life have created the unfolding
of today's circumstances. The new world calls for us to live
from a foundation of presence, so we are awake to focus on
our expansion. As we focus on expansion, we expand. As we
expand, we become expanded beings with expanded minds and
move away from the limited thinking of the ego.

Mastery itself is a moment-to-moment process lived through
a new worldview. It is an unfolding of ourselves back to our
most basic state of allowing, where we can live consciously in
the direction of our dreams. Nothing to fret about if this seems
like a far cry from where you are now. The path will meet you
where you are today; I'm just telling you about the good stuff
coming.

Awake athletes will experience mindset shifts that induce
irrevocable personal transformation because once we supersede
self-induced suffering, we will never go back to the old world

way of being. Anchor yourself, though, because it takes nothing less than repetitive practice over a long period of time. That said, you will feel benefits immediately. Even the messiest meditations will further attune you to the limitlessness of your source.

The new worldview embraces all experiences as learning opportunities. Even the darkest days are seen from a solution-oriented view because, as deliberate co-creators, we know that the problem expands if we focus on the problem. If we focus on the solution, the solution expands. And although the problem and solution are born simultaneously, they cannot co-exist. We cannot find a solution in the energy of a problem.

Often when BJ is on the phone with an athlete he coaches who is struggling, I'll hear him say, "Can we agree that what you've been doing is not working for what you want to achieve?" Only when he and the athlete reach this agreement can he begin assisting them toward a solution for their problem. I inevitably hear him direct the conversation away from whatever limits the athlete and move the conversation toward what the athlete can do to continue creating momentum toward their goal. The two of them progress from obstacle to potential and what most people may miss here is that the open-minded nature of the conversation alone helps the athlete move towards their goal.

It's the old world way to scrutinize what is wrong. Many of us are trying to figure out the problem instead of welcoming a solution. Seeking the guidance of a teacher or coach queued into a new worldview is critical to swiftly getting out of the problem and repatterning your brain to a new world default. But it's important to remember that the teacher or coach is simply the pointer. You must be willing to see your life situation through the eyes of possibility. As you do this, with time, you will see that every bit of your experience is valuable, even the contrast. Because, with contrast, we have the opportunity to strengthen our desire to go after what we want. Joy and challenge hold equal value to an awake athlete.

When BJ and I settled into our life here in California and went full bore into creating the community and coaching business of YogiTriathlete, we were first met with the response of crickets. The stream of financial abundance flowed in drips, not floods, and we were running out of money quickly, but the purpose driving us forward far exceeded material evidence, and that could not be denied. We had to keep going. Sure, we feared financial ruin, but we did not buy into those thoughts. We were too far down the road to believe in lack as truth. Clearly, we were receiving an opportunity to burn the karma that brought us to these challenges. We stood surefooted under the guidance of our teacher to welcome all that was coming our way. We had entered the world of debt before and come out of it and were entering it again, but this time with a commitment to viewing it differently.

We developed an abundance mindset, not just around money but in a way where we were building the business for the good of all. And when we surrendered to the circumstances, we gained the power of focus and vision to see that it was all happening for us, not to us. When we step into our days with a new worldview, we are apt to lay down our arms of defense and release the fight against what life is unfolding. Only then can we appreciate the value of all that comes our way. When we decide to take back our power by being in charge of our response, we can relax into the feelings that arise and see the meaning we are giving those moments of life. We tend to put more importance on some things than others, but yoga would say that every moment is just as important as the next. The moment you came into the world and the moment you picked up your toothbrush this morning are equally worthy.

During my yoga teacher training, I learned that everything is inherently neutral until we give it meaning. Much of the meaning we give causes deep suffering in our lives. The mind constantly labels life as right or wrong, good or bad, and it has been doing that unsupervised for a long time. By social conditioning, most of us attune to old world separatism and modern-day negativity. These unhelpful neural pathways are so well-paved that it could take the rest of your life to starve them of energy, so right now is the best time to start.

It would be best to decide that as you pay attention to your life that you'll be gentle with yourself when you are stewing in problem energy. Gentleness is at the core of our power to change because gentle energy aligns with calm energy, and calm energy aligns with source energy. Have you noticed that no detail was left undone in the beauty of nature or the body's intelligence? Creation is not hectic energy; it does not rush or skip steps but always accomplishes everything.

Once we attune to calm, the conscious choice becomes our least-action pathway. This is powerful living from a new worldview, and it is dependent on our ability to make good on our decision not to stay the same. As long as we are paying attention, we will learn when we are indulging a resistant perspective and when we are indulging an acceptance perspective. The fight associated with resistance is the marrow of our constriction in life. When an electrical wire has resistance, the flow of electricity is compromised; when we lessen the resistance, more electricity flows. Same here; when we reduce the resistance to how life flows, we open to the current of life. It's impossible to be disconnected from the cosmic force, but when we resist its stream, we feel less of its supportive power. Over time, higher resistance means lower feelings of trust and faith. We fight because we have no clue how much we are loved and held by something bigger than we know. But as we lessen our resistance, we will feel more of that something bigger.

A new worldview is expansive and limitless, so we must release our constrictions to open up and live in the new world. The first recognition of your desire to live with a new worldview is letting go of the belief that what we see, hear, taste, touch, and smell is all there is. There is non-physical support that is always with you. Most of you are not tapping into it, and when you do, it is usually in the form of desperate pleas and awkward conversations that start, "Hi God, I know we do not talk very often..." I know, I've been there, and it always felt icky. Like I was a less-than-being begging from another I felt unworthy of, so most of the time, I avoided that being altogether. As a result, I buried myself in the maya of this physical world, which outside of dogma, does not educate us to develop a relationship with the non-physical.

This world of physicality is dense and obvious. The world of non-physicality is neither; it's subtle and limitless. To the conditioned mind and the ego, the unknown of limitlessness is scary. Our nervous systems perceive the unknown as a threat, so we easily catastrophize minor things, transforming them into big things. Next thing you know, we have school yards that look like prison yards and people who are too afraid to ride their bikes on the road. We have welcomed fear into our lives, and it has manifested in so many different forms; anxiety, anger, sadness, worry, and loneliness, to name a few. All it breeds is more of the same. It denies our universal connection and leads to a scarcity mindset. It is old world living where we invite what we do not want into our lives. And if you look closely at the foundation of society, you will see all the calling cards of an old world mind. It's no wonder we ended up here.

The new worldview understands that intent is the seed of creation, and when we focus on and act from intent, we open space for the universe to do the heavy lifting on our behalf. Fear is fueled by the feeling we have lost control, and this feels powerless, which makes us cling tighter. As we connect with universal energy through our practices, we naturally trust more because we are tuned to its immense power.

This is available to everyone. It's otherworldly, yet it is within you right now. It's the one unchanging reality in a world that is always changing, and it sits at the base of all life. Scientists have studied the smallest subatomic particles and continue to seek the core entity. Like Einstein, who held one goal, to understand the unity that underlies the diversity of nature, science continues to seek the God particle. Still, they will never find it because it is everything. It is the source of all that science has discovered and has yet to uncover. It's the unknown, the unobvious. The manifest and unmanifest. The time-space reality where all possibilities live.

We live in what I've heard termed a holographic reality, a three-dimensional light field. When our bodies and minds dwell only in 3D, we are not open to experiencing the many other dimensions that exist for us to experience. The stillness of meditation attunes us to higher frequencies, weakening our reliance on the dense energy of the 3D field. If we remain steadfast in our practice, we will experience what quantum physics calls zero-state awareness or, as yoga says, a state of no mind. The state where time is lost. It's sitting for a 30-minute meditation that feels like a moment or two. It is the unification of all things, the nature of a new worldview realized when we commit to sit and recondition our mind through a steadfast meditation practice.

CHAPTER FIVE

COMMIT TO SIT

"If one does not stay committed, one will never grow."

Meditator Bob

Legs crossed, hips elevated, sacrum aligned with the top of my head. Mala beads in hand; I am ready to meditate. The gong sounds three times from the meditation timer on my phone. I begin my practice.

I open my body to gravity and envision a healing light coming up from the earth and into my feet. Slowly it engulfs my entire body in a protective shield, healing bodily niggles[8] along the way and increasing my ability to adapt to the stresses of my training load. I picture the light exiting the crown of my head, moving through the ceiling, and beyond the clouds. It surpasses the atmosphere and fades into the abyss of the universe. I am

8 Niggle is a common term used in endurance athletics to describe an area of the body where someone is experiencing persistent yet slight discomfort.

open to the field.

I silently recite a mantra to concentrate and calm the mind 108 times as I slide my fingers from one rudraksha bead to the next. I practice kriya[9] while focusing on the space in the middle of my forehead, just above my eyebrows. And then, I move into silent meditation.

"Those kriyas were good today."

"I wonder how much time I have left."

"Shit, I'm meditating."

"Don't think the word shit when you are meditating."

I redirect my focus to the mantra, so hum.

"I must get back to Gail about the podcast."

"Why do I always remember everything when I'm meditating?"

"I wish I could take notes."

Soooo Hummm.

"I will remember everything that I'm supposed to."

Soooo Hummm.

9 Kriya is a yoga practice centered around breath control.

I churn within the cyclical nature of neural loops over and over like a hamster on a wheel. When I wake up and find myself in the circus of my mind, I bring my attention back to the moment but inevitably, I drift again. Sometimes I drift into states of no mind and sometimes into wondrous visions, but often it's a straight shot into the irrelevant goings-on of my mind. And yet, despite the commotion, I stay the course.

I return to the meditation cushion daily because it is a practice, and I am an athlete. Training the mind is just like training the body. Consistency is everything to my success. Sometimes it is a fiasco, but it is never a waste. My commitment to sit has yielded me a better life. I am different now. I am lighter, not so serious, and hard-lined. My relationship with everything from family to food, training, and racing has undeniably transformed for the better. This is because meditation is like filling an ice cube tray. Start with one corner and let the water flow; eventually, it serves every part of the tray.

On paper, my meditations appear skillful. If someone were to walk in and see me sitting still on my cushion with nag champa incense burning in a tray beside me, they might think I have mastered this whole meditation thing. But appearances are deceiving, and they do not see the familiar battle waging under the facade. Although there are many stretches of actual meditation these days, most of the time, I practice dharana, not dhyana. And my ego hates that you know that about me.

Within the limbs of yoga, concentration precedes meditation. It is what most athletes do when they sit for meditation practice and is an essential precursor to entering states of meditation. When we practice concentration, we use techniques like mantra and pranayama, tools like mala beads and candle flames to concentrate the mind so that the monkey slows its swing, and we can enter the state of meditation. These practices tune us to the quiet within by making the mind one-pointed. So it's not about creating quiet; it's tuning to the quiet already within us despite the activity of thoughts. A belief derailing many is that they are not meditating the right way. Yes, there are techniques, but the abiding truth is your inner being knows how to meditate. It is the essence of meditation; it's the very being you meet in meditation.

When you commit to sit, you will discover this part of you, the awake athlete within. I promise you it's there right now, patiently waiting. I've found it, and many athletes I work with have also seen it. The following story is one example of many I have heard over the years and one that I don't expect will ever get old.

After two years of working together, one of my clients told me she felt her inner being for the first time during meditation. She called it her core. This awake athlete is a highly intellectual, well-accomplished competitor who had been battling meditation for the better of those two years. And that day, she said she found something "underneath it all" and recognized it as herself.

"Is that me?" she asked.

"Yes," I replied, "that's you."

Like many of us do, this athlete was judging her practice daily. Her intellect was taking score, and she was commonly frustrated by the lack of evidence that she was successful. But she stayed committed despite all the noise. She never wavered in her consistency to sit every day, something that I find common among highly motivated athletes. She knew she had to get through the loud parts to attune to the quiet within.

At the time of her discovery, we were focusing on relaxing techniques like slowing down her breath in times of frustration. She was aware that she was fighting the meditation, and she was ready to let go of the battle. Through breath control, she began to allow that fight to fall away, clearing space for her to experience her core Self.

This is available to all of us, and with consistency, you will also live it. But only with consistency because that is what keeps the mind strong. When we don't train our bodies, we lose fitness. The same goes for the mind. We have to chop the wood and carry the water. We must shovel the hay into the barn, and yoga teaches us how to do it all with the necessary grace of patience.

When MB told me that patience attains the goal, I knew I had a mountain to climb. I was not skilled at being patient. In truth, I revered my impatience. I thought it was a strength, but now I know it is not, and my performance suffered more than a few times because of my impatience.

One time that stands out is when we were living in Boulder and I adopted the Metabolic Aerobic Function (MAF)[10] method for training. This method can be a nightmare for the impatient ones, and that was me. I know many of you have tried MAF, and in that case, I bet you fall into one of two camps:

1) You tried it, didn't work (impatience).
2) You now run faster paces at your MAF heart rate (patience).

The practice of meditation is much the same. Those who try it will typically land in one of those two camps, and it's important to know that both have value. Camp two for obvious reasons but also camp one because it was here that you planted seeds of change. And because it is our nature to grow and expand, you will inevitably receive opportunities to water those seeds throughout your life.

Regarding my MAF training experience, I fell into camp one for many years. This was during the early 2000s when the mind was still in charge of me, and it appeared that everyone but me who tried MAF found success. This triggered stories of unworthiness for me. These stories said that I was already slow and getting slower because I was attempting to run at a lower heart rate and nothing seemed to change. Running so slow hurt and biking so slow meant I would be alone for the rest of my life. I had so many reasons to stop, and in the end, I allowed discouragement to win. So I quit, and I wasn't faster. It would be almost two decades before I watered my seeds and

10 MAF is the method of Metabolic Aerobic Function, a technique of training the body exclusively under a certain heart rate or beats per minute (BPM) to build aerobic fitness. One can find their MAF number by subtracting their age from the number 180.

recommitted to MAF training.

It happened in the summer of 2020 when it became apparent
I needed to take a break from running. I sustained an injury in
my right foot that seemingly came out of nowhere and hung
around for several months. I had just completed the Bryce
Canyon 50-miler when the sensation showed up, a point in the
center of my right heel that felt like I was struck by a flaming
arrow. Running was off the table entirely, and walking was far
from sensation-free. The problem was apparent, and I could see
that I needed to tune myself to the solution, or I would prolong
my path to recovery.

I made a list in my journal about everything I could do and
started with the top three: swim, bike, and meditate more.
After that, I upped my game in the pool, bought a bike, and
dedicated myself to MAF training while spending more time
on the meditation cushion. The results of my recommitment to
MAF showed within the first few months, and when I got back
to running, they translated. I look back now and contribute
most of this success not with time in the workouts but in the
time clearing my mental clutter over the years. It becomes
easier to yield to the benefits of life experience with patience, as
the mental obstacles to patience dissipate through our commit
to sit practice.

In this particular instance of injury, the light shined bright on
three significant benefits: 1) returning to MAF training allowed
me to become a fitter, more efficient athlete while healing, 2)
it drove me to start riding again, which sparked a joy I had yet

to feel in my relationship with the bike and 3) it got me back into triathlon, fulfilling a desire to have it all; training for trail running and triathlon.

Had I chosen to stay in the problem of that injury, I would have increased focus on the pain, the sadness of not running, and the depressive energy that comes when we feel like we are being held back. I would have never found the joy that was an instant away at all times. And I never would have known about the joy if I had not experienced the benefits of slowing down over the years through the patient practice of meditation and yoga. I have witnessed the stillness behind every thought and beneath every heartbeat. It is the base of all that is true, and it never leaves you—not during a sprint finish, a relentless climb, an injury, DNF[11], a divorce, or death. It's rooted in patience, found in presence, and boundless in its love for all beings and all circumstances. It is layers deep, but it is there nonetheless.

Meditation offers us a front-row seat to the action of the mind and shows us where our mind is dwelling so that we can begin to move through the layers holding us from our truth and potential. Once we see where our mind dwells, we can stay or pivot at any moment. After a while in your practice, you will quickly catch yourself when you are complaining, gossiping, or participating in other less-than-desirable behaviors and act on your power to pivot focus. You will choose breath awareness in the face of lower self noise. You will decide to feel your feet in your shoes or think of something you are grateful for in

---

11 DNF is an acronym for Did Not Finish and is listed next to the athlete's name at the end of the official results listing.

moments of overwhelm and stress. You will choose to give your fuel to anything but the tantrum of your mind once you realize that you are in charge of your mental dwelling place.

Outside circumstances are constantly changing; nothing ever stays the same. We live in an ocean of motion where the only certainty is uncertainty. But when we develop a relationship with ourselves through sitting practice, we feel less shaky when the earth and its beings tremble. It doesn't matter what is happening outside of you because you will be familiar with your power to choose the response that continually guides you to the life you desire. Being awake does not make you immune to receiving lower self impulses like impatience, greed, or doubt. It just means that you'll be able to notice those moments and see them for what they are, moments of contrast where you have a choice. Since there is plenty of contrast to experience each day, you will also begin to notice that humans are quite drunk on the drama of life, and they cannot see that all they have to do is put the bottle down. There is an addiction to negative thoughts, causing many to suffer greatly.

In *Bhagavad Gita: As It Is* Swami Prabhupada describes this earth as a land of misery, and we are here to overcome it. We have allowed misery to rule our lives at different junctures, but when we decide that it will be no longer, we open to its opposite—joy. Sometimes the journey is painless, sometimes painful, traumatic even, but it doesn't matter how we get to any particular moment. The only direction is forward, and how we move forward matters most because that vibration maps our future. The more clarity and control we have over our minds, the stronger our ability to deliberately create our lives. Patanjali describes the mind as a veil of thoughts that blocks our inner light; for most, that veil is a dense organism. Meditation thins the veil as it teaches us to watch our thoughts.

Like a heap of sugar, if we pull away each grain, there will be a point when there is no sugar. We diminish the heap as we notice our thoughts, allow them to pass through, and consciously choose how to move forward in a moment. We loosen the fabric, and the veil thins. As the veil thins, we open to enlightened perspectives that welcome us to a powerful journey forward.

To receive this invitation to ultimate success, we must turn away from excuses that keep us the same by being open to shifting bad habits while adopting good ones. Chances are, your meditation practice will not be pretty for a while. You will have the temptation to skip your practice, and you will succumb. You will tell yourself that you'll do it later, and not until the next day will you realize that you never made it to the cushion. Your mind will be busy, and it will be tempting to quit, but do not quit. You are entering a state of change, and there will be resistance. Sit anyway. Sit despite your busy mind, and sit to calm your nervous system. Sit because you can, and sit to get to know the thoughts dictating your reality.

The practice of meditation creates a deeper relationship with ourselves. The one we think we know but don't, and the one we need to know to live fully. It is the subtle part of us resting behind the thought forms; the Seer. We catch glimpses of it in the space between the thoughts, and the yogis also call it the witness Self. I call it the unshakeable Self. It is the part of us we can only experience, and we do that by turning our awareness inward through meditation and practicing its corresponding limbs—pranayama (breath control), pratyahara (sense control), etc. These practices firm up our foundation so that the base of what drives us forward is solid, and when we are honest with ourselves, we will see that an unshakeable foundation serves our endeavors best.

I lived through grave resistance from my ego to sit in silence and turn my focus inward. Like many, an addiction to *doing* kept me from contentment and peace and in the limited mindset of excuses for years. Even though I always carried a positive attitude, external circumstances heavily influenced its steadiness. When my boat got rocked, I lost my peace, and my ego ensured there was carnage in my wake. Through blame and victimhood, I was bound and determined to take others down with me. By keeping busy, I buried my head in accomplishment and turned a blind eye to my shaky foundation. I can now see the falsehood of believing meditation was not for me because I was too good at *doing*. Feeling productive was my meditation, running was my meditation, everything but stillness was my meditation, even drinking wine.

I never thought much about my inability to sit still until one afternoon in our home on Darley Avenue in Boulder. I completed my to-dos for the day, so I walked around the house a bit, straightening things until nothing was left to straighten. I decided to sit down with nothing else; no laptop, phone, nothing. Just me, sitting in my living room, attempting to do what I had seen others do in boho lifestyle magazines. It was no big deal in my mind at the time. However, when my body hit the couch, I immediately ejected to a vertical position and found myself staring into a mirror, literally and figuratively. I saw every stressed, overworked, overactive person I ever gossiped about staring back at me. It saw my inner world. Front and center with no to-do to cover it up.

Divine intervention? Yes, indeed. A moment of awakening? Absolutely.

At the time, I considered myself deep into a holistic way of life, a shift accelerated by contracting West Nile Virus in 2003, which woke me up to the profound benefits of homeopathy and acupuncture. I was no stranger to energy work, local and non-local craniosacral therapy sessions, a ten-series of structural integration, or weekly massages. Psychic readings, past-life regression, ayahuasca, and boiling twigs on the stovetop to heal bones and increase my blood volume were never off the table. I assure you I was well into mellowing out but still, I was not attending to my mind.

One would think this moment of clarity in my living room was when I committed to sit, but it would be several years before I started my meditation practice. Nevertheless, the clarity I experienced that day never diminished, and I noticed my resistance to being in silence with myself. When I found my way to the cushion years later, it was in the silence that I felt my impatience, my judgments, and my jealousy. I saw her again, my shadow self. She was still alive, and I identified her as the source of all stress and unhappiness in my life. She was the same girl I saw that day in the mirror. No wonder life sometimes felt so hard, and people were jerks. All the struggles I experienced in the outside world were not outside of me. As long as I stayed surface, looking to others for my healing and pointing fingers at others for my relief, I did not see my undesirables. And when I did, it was not easy to see, and it may not be easy for you, no matter how positive your attitude may be. But when we are willing to see and feel ourselves move through the world, we can change what we see is not benefiting ourselves, our communities, our performance, and our dreams.

Meditation teaches us to observe debilitating mental mechanisms, like negative neural loops, which easily get covered up when we are constantly *on the go*. As we recognize the non-serving nature of specific thoughts and patterns, we can focus on the present moment, where we are at our best. Presence is a muscle that builds over time, and it is the body-mind intersection where epic performances live. Over twenty years ago, it was concluded that present moment focus is the essence of the psychology of peak performance in sport (Jackson & Csikszentmihalyi, 1999; Ravizza, 2002). It is well-said that competition is 90% mental and 10% physical, so nothing would be more wasteful than neglecting an opportunity to strengthen an athlete's mind. I have practiced yoga for almost three decades, and I started my endurance life in 2005—my meditation practice in 2010. My experience is that nothing builds the mental acuity needed for high-pressure situations and times of duress more than meditation.

There is a wealth of scientific studies showing that mindfulness and meditation affect gray matter in the brain. More gray matter means more brain connectivity. For example, in a study out of Harvard University (Holzel, Lazar, et al. 2011), daily Mindfulness-Based Stress Reduction (MBSR) meditation showed changes in the brain after just eight weeks. Areas of the brain related to muscle control, perception, body awareness, pain tolerance, and regulation of emotions, particularly resiliency, were strengthened. I would expect that resiliency is of great interest to you as it determines ability to roll with the punches. Learning to experience life in a non-resistant manner allows us to overcome mental obstacles like how hard it is to meditate. A study by the University of Wisconsin concluded, "A meditation habit can strengthen the body's immune function, plus increase brain performance in the form of electrical activity." During meditation, blood flow increases, and heart rate balances, enhancing the immune system. Shifts like these heal the body and mind so we can continue to train and experience longevity in our sport.

A meditative mind also helps us hone our skills of discernment and intuition. As a result, we will better know when to push through and when to back off. Like the other limbs of yoga, meditation shines a light on our physical and mental weak spots before they fully bloom into illness, injury or disease. I am not promising that meditation nullifies injury because it does not, and sometimes what is best for our growth will come from illness or injury. However, if we can use those experiences to watch for victim-like perspectives and focus on honing our response, we will consciously direct our momentum forward. I often discuss injury on the Awake Athlete podcast, so tune in for companion material to this book.

Are you convinced to commit to sit yet? Or do you still believe that running is meditation? Because it is not. Meditation is not movement. Moving meditation is movement. What I'm talking about is stillness. And if it feels too far a distance to venture, know that the only way we can adapt to stillness is to practice being still, and you can start right now with one breath. Every conscious breath counts. One breath is a planted seed. So contrary to beliefs that you must be a full renunciate of the material world and live in a cave in the Himalayas, anyone can dive into meditation at any time.

There will be times, especially at first, when the thoughts in your mind are on a death march to kill your silence. For some of you, this will happen often. My first year of meditation was a street fight, a break-the-neck-off a beer bottle fight. Somedays, I sat with my eyes closed and screamed. I kid you not, I can only imagine what my neighbors heard, but I had stuffed my emotional vault for so many years that I felt like a tea kettle overboiling on the stove. My nervous system was a mess even though I believed I was not a stressed person, at least not all the time. And this is the case for most of you. It's okay; this is not a judgment. It is the state of affairs. Our society lives in fight or flight, and we will continue to live in fight or flight if we identify with the external world as our primary reality. The World Health Organization called stress the "health epidemic of the 21st century." Stress is at the core of dis-ease and imbalance in the body and mind. Studies on meditation and mindfulness show, and participants report, significant decreases in stress from practicing meditation. Stillness activates the body's healing mechanisms and shifts our rest and digest parasympathetic nervous system (PNS) into gear—a balanced nervous system aids in systematically reducing stress and inflammation.

Considering the world we live in and the *go, go, go* mentality, it should be no surprise that when we first sit down to meditate, it can feel like trying to stop a blender with our tongue. The idea of achieving no mind in the first few hundred tries brought me to the brink more than a few times, but the willingness to go back time and time again ultimately made the difference. Every time we sit for meditation, our brains react by building gray matter in areas that benefit our performance, relationships, and, most importantly, how we respond to the world around us. Before I started meditating, I considered sitting still by myself in silence while holding my athletic body in an uncomfortable posture, a living hell in the comfort of my home. It was the absolute last thing I ever planned to do in this life, yet undeniably, there had always been a voice inside me that called for stillness. This voice is the exact piece of you that is gaining a more robust flavor in your life. I know this because you would not be reading this sentence if you were not already waking up. So, what keeps you from knowing yourself better so you can be better?

Athletes desire betterment for themselves, and athletic potential requires the same. Yet, we are so good at neglecting the mind when everyone knows that the mind is where the difference is made. It is not more complicated than sitting down, shutting your mouth, closing your eyes, and not moving for a series of moments each day. Living as an awake athlete is the most natural thing, yet such an unexpected turn in my journey. I never planned to meditate, but since committing to sit, I have realized that it is why I came here to this earth, and because you are still here with me on this page, I think it may be a part of your journey too.

CHAPTER SIX

TAME THE MIND

"The mind is restless, turbulent, powerful, violent;
trying to control it is like trying to tame the wind."

Bhagavad Gita

Clark is our golden retriever. He is six years old as I write this
line. His addition to our family did not fit the plan, but here
he is, lying at my feet. Much like meditation, Clark was a
gift in our lives that I did not know we needed at the time of
his arrival. It had been a decade since BJ, and I were puppy
parents, and from Clark's first tear through the house, it was
clear we had grown accustomed to the tame life of senior dogs.

On his first night home, I took him outside into the freezing
Rhode Island air. Our ice-laden driveway reflected the
moonlight like a mirror. Back and forth, Clark ran with more
speed and strength than I had seen in a long time, especially
for such a small package. He was wiping out and getting back
up repeatedly with an unbridled enthusiasm that felt as fun as

it did frightening. There was no safety net with Clark, and I found a deep sense of freedom as I observed him engage in a boundaryless relationship with joy.

I met Clark's soul in those moments on that brisk night. He called me into his presence and easily kept me there with his ridiculously adorable 12-week-old golden retriever body. His fur was as white as a polar bear, and his muscles surprisingly developed. Clark's joy was so unbound that it changed me in an instant. I absorbed his rowdy character and glimpsed the handsome boy he has since grown to become. He exuded silliness that I had not felt in years. I knew he was our teacher, but we were to teach him first. Training would be vital for Clark and us to thrive as a family. And so structured with clear boundaries, loving reinforcement, and victorious celebrations, we grew over time into the bonded pack we are today.

On his second day at home, I returned from teaching a yoga class and sat with him for over an hour on the kitchen floor. Him sleeping on my lap, and me just being. I noticed a level of contentment that did not allow me to get up and move forward in my day. Of course, my mind initially spun out about everything I needed to get done that day, but as I stayed, all that clutter fell away. He drew me into a state of presence, and I was tame to it.

I would have entertained the mind in past frequencies and denied the bonding experience in front of me. But I've learned that as we yoke the mind every day to be with us in stillness, we are more apt to get yoked into other present moment experiences. And just as Clark taught me to sit and stay that day, and I went on to teach him the same a thousand times, we can also do this with our minds. But to be successful, we must have a toolbox of mind training techniques. Concrete methods that give the mind something to do while we learn to direct it toward the desired behavior. This is the same recipe BJ and I used to train Clark.

Tools are particularly helpful in getting the mind on board with your commitment to sit and live awake because it loves to feel productive. By employing techniques, you're tasking the mind instead of the mind tasking you. You are instructing the mind from present-moment awareness to engage in thinking and acting on your behalf.

The most effective tactics we learned when training Clark was never to use the word "no" and to never punish him. Instead, our trainer helped us redirect him toward the desired behavior and then trained us to celebrate the victory with him. She helped us see that "no" was the problem. "No" referred to what we did not want, and in doing so, we received more of what we did not want. Of course, it was the problem. This makes so much sense. Who would have guessed it? Our dog trainer was teaching us quantum physics, and our unplanned puppy was the catalyst.

Everything we taught Clark translates to mind training. Interrupt the behavior and gently redirect. Celebrate your victories by allowing yourself to feel the peace they render and stay focused on what you want. As I said, clear boundaries, loving reinforcement, and victorious celebrations. It worked like a charm for Clark, and it works like a charm for the mind while it also aligns us with ahimsa. It allows us to do the least harm because we never punish ourselves, our puppies, or anyone again.

Just like Clark needed a hierarchy established, the mind also needs a commanding presence to thrive. And that commanding presence must be you. Tools and techniques give it something to chew on, so the monkey slows its swing, and the puppy stops peeing in the house. The tools and techniques that I offer in this book are simple. Spirituality is simple. Living awake is simple, but we live in a world obsessed with over-complication and over-intellectualization, which keeps us under the mind's rule. Techniques and tools are used to train the mind to interrupt these patterns and give us space to choose desired behaviors consciously. The two most potent in my training are breath and mantra. With earnest effort in practice, they are all we ever need.

BREATH

Let's look at this epic tool of all time for all humankind, the breath. Every being has it, and it's automatic, but when we step in and make it deliberate, we change everything about our experience and how our bodies and minds can accept a moment.

Ujjayi Breath

This style of breath is a yogic breath that flows in and out through the nose. It is often first learned in an asana class setting, but it is a breath that is helpful in many other areas of life. I learned this style by breathing in through my nose and breathing out through my mouth. As I exhaled, I held my palm in front of my mouth and breathed out as if I was fogging a mirror. Give it a try, and notice the natural constriction in the back of your throat when you fog the mirror. It is the same constriction felt when whispering, so give that some practice too. After a while, close your mouth, keep the constriction in your throat and exhale through your nose. Continue breathing in and out through the nose. Ujjayi breath is a controlled, audible breath whereby we do not gulp or dump the air as it enters and exits our system. It's a way of breathing that produces equanimity no matter the circumstance. I highly recommend you master it.

Conscious Breathing
One conscious breath can shift the world. So if that is all you are willing to experience in a day, start each day with one mindful breath and know that you are contributing to a better world. In that one breath, you are accessing your best self and offering your best energy to the world because in that breath you are present.

There are many ways to take a conscious breath; the following is one variation; the only requirement of mindful breathing is your full attention. Let's take one together right now.

1) Take a long slow breath through your nose (ujjayi would work great here). Shoot for a count of four or six. Fill until you feel a gentle pressure in your chest and lungs.

2) Hold your breath in for a count of four.

3) Calmly breathe out, extending the exhale longer than your inhale, a count of eight to 12. Our parasympathetic nervous system governs exhalation, so by breathing out longer, you activate the PNS, which is a good thing because it helps us experience rest and healing.

4) Hold your breath out until you feel the impulse to breathe in again.

5) Then slowly, watch for gulping, refill with air and resume normal breathing.

As we consciously breathe daily, we open to more pauses. This leads us to the always profound space where we may entertain a new worldview if we have fallen into the old world. And we will fall because it's normal for the mind to fall throughout our day, but a new perspective brings a refreshed frequency, leaving unhelpful tendencies unfed. As layers that no longer serve us disband through energetic starvation, we recondition our minds. As we deliberately recondition the mind, we tame the mind. For this process, I find breath to be a perfect tool.

Breath is also the most powerful interface to our nervous system. Suppose you are prone to overwhelm, panic, jealousy, judgment, low self-worth, or any of the million other symptoms of stress. In that case, you can utilize breath to concentrate the mind and create physiological changes in your body. Exercises involving breath can energize, calm and balance your entire body and mind.

Remember, this is pranayama, the fourth limb of the supreme science. Pranayama translates to life force management which we do through our breath. The self-regulation from practicing pranayama elicits positive change and desirable motion forward in your life. Whenever you recognize a pattern of behavior or neural loop you no longer desire to indulge in, you can interrupt the cycle by shifting your awareness to the breath. Of course, conscious breathing does not mean the chatter will subside, but it does mean you are taking control of your mind, introducing change, and no longer fueling what you do not want.

For race performance, pranayama pays a premium to the awake athlete. Like many seasoned athletes, I've learned the hard way and worked back from there. I know how it feels to have tight breathing muscles before a race that quickly leads to feeling like I cannot get a breath. During a triathlon swim, this can mean a panic attack in the water. For a trail race or cycling event, this can mean exerting gratuitous effort and falling off pace quickly. Many times I have turned my head to breathe while swimming and got a mouthful of water or a fist in my face. Being calm enough to skip a breath while being punched in the face, or the like for a runner, is crucial to remaining in control during a physically challenging experience.

The following is a breakdown of pranayama exercises that have proven successful for numerous athletes. Many have said that these breathing techniques saved their race-day performance. So give them a try at your next starting line, presentation, confrontation, or anything that puts you out of your comfort zone. Also, practice them at the beginning of your daily meditation; they are great for calming the body and concentrating the mind.

Three-Part Breath

1) Breathe into your belly, and feel it expand. Pause, don't exhale. Breathe into your lungs and feel the expansion of your ribs. Pause, don't exhale. Breathe into your chest and feel your collarbone lift.

2) Pause at the top of the breath, then exhale slowly.

3) Repeat three times using nostril breathing.

Breathe of Fire

1) Start with a cleansing breath through your nose and out through your mouth.

2) Breathe in through your nose, and without pausing, exhale forcefully through your nose by pumping your low belly inward. The inhale should feel automatic as you solely focus on the exhale. Practice several times, then speed it up—the breath should be quick and loud. Start with a count of 15-20; over time, build up to 30-45 as you master this technique.

3) After the last breath, inhale deeply, hold the breath in and lock your pelvic floor muscles and imagine an upward trajectory of your energy. Hold until you have the impulse to

breathe, then slowly exhale through your nose or mouth.

4) Repeat three times.

Tense and Release
1) Take a big nostril breath in and tense every muscle in your body. Do not hurt yourself, but tense everything: toes, heels, shins, calf muscles, hamstrings, quads, belly, ribs, heart, lungs, arms, fingers, neck, face, and everything in between.

2) Hold for five seconds.

3) Then release through your mouth, emptying your body and squeezing all the air out of your lungs.

4) Repeat three times.

Relaxing Breath
1) Breathe in through your nose for a count of four.

2) Hold for a count of seven.

3) Exhale through your nose for a count of eight.

4) Repeat three times.

This breath has kicked up feelings of anxiety for some athletes. If this is the case for you, start with an inhale of two and an exhale of four. You can build from there or try this breath without the seven-count hold. Many times that will do the trick.

Alternate Nostril Breathing

1) Place your right thumb on your right nostril and fold in your index and middle finger.

2) Inhale through your left nostril.

3) Once you inhale completely, put your ring finger over your left nostril, release your right nostril and breathe out.

4) Inhale through the right nostril.

5) Once you inhale completely, put your thumb over your right nostril, release your left nostril and breathe out. That is one complete cycle.

6) Inhale through your left nostril and repeat the steps above.

7) Complete three sets of three.

Breathe Less

On average, we take 25,000 breaths daily, and there is evidence that breathing less is better. James Nestor's book *Breath: The New Science Of A Lost Art* reports the optimal breathing pattern is 5.5 nasal breaths per minute. This pace of breath creates an optimal level of CO_2 in the body, which maximizes oxygen absorption. Like resiliency, this factoid should be of particular interest to all athletes.

So, throughout your day, notice your breath and ask yourself if you can breathe less. Slow down your breath and notice the pause between each breath. Notice the moments when the inhale turns into the exhale and the exhale into the inhale. Then shape your breath to be smooth, devoid of choppiness or rough spots. Like pouring oil into oil, make your breath seamless. Time yourself and see how many breaths you usually take per minute, then shoot for 5.5 nasal breaths. Notice the difference. Also, practice nasal breathing during aerobic workouts (MAF) to keep your pace honest and your heart rate low.

MANTRA

A mantra is a word, sound, or statement repeated to concentrate the mind and tune it to a desired frequency (i.e., calm, grateful, confident, and so on). Athletes have been using mantras for ages, and material science backs their efficacy. However, yogis take the practice of mantras further and use them to etch positive grooves within one's consciousness and heal negative grooves. These grooves are impressions of our past actions, known as samskaras.

Samskaras are something we accumulate over the long journey of life. We bring them into this world through our soul body, and they can be both positive and negative. The positive ones are our natural talents and gifts, selfless service, loving kindness; they help us evolve. In contrast, negative samskaras get in the way of our evolution. They are what we need to overcome to become masters of our minds and realize our true Self. By repeating and feeling the vibration of a mantra in practice, we can positively affect our negative samskaras and move past the distortion they create. There is no better time for these samskaras to shine than when we are physically fatigued and broken down by stress. Racing is the perfect example of when we may feel the influence of our negative etchings and mantra is an effective way to put the brakes on their expansion.

The following mantras are some of my favorites. I have found them all extra helpful in taming the mind in training, racing, and life, especially when it feels like the wheels are falling off in training, racing and life.

So hum

So hum is known as a universal mantra, meaning anyone can use it regardless of their belief or faith. It resonates as the vibration of peace and is said to match the natural sounds of the breath. When concentrated upon, we can hear the syllable *so* as we inhale and *hum* as we exhale. The translation of this mantra is, "I am that I am." Yoga scholars interpret "that" as the universal energy we are connected to and the one that nourishes us with precisely what we need. Repeat the word *soooo* on the inhale and *hummm* on the exhale to activate its resonance. As you feel the vibration, you imprint your subconscious with the very essence that holds the universe together as one.

I'm fine, right now, I'm fine

This mantra was helpful in the early stages of my meditation practice as I experienced significant anxiety rise from within me. It allowed me to feel what I needed to let go of without identifying with stories projecting from the past onto the feeling. This is a clean way to let go—feel without identifying with the whirlpool of thoughts or vritti. I also found this quite helpful when I first embarked on the trails by myself and faced the fears that kept me from trail running for years and during triathlon swims when panic arrived at my door because it kept me in the now where I could see I was just that—absolutely fine.

I can do miraculous things with very little effort

I once carried the perspective that I had to do everything throughout my life because no one would do it if I didn't. And if they did, it wouldn't be right. So this mantra was quite helpful in releasing the self-induced burdens that I carried during even the smallest of tasks, and it freed me from the victimhood that kept me in moments of powerless misery. It further awakened me to my divine essence, the energy that makes all things possible. Also, one should not underestimate this mantra's power during the marathon of a long distance triathlon, ultra-endurance race, or endeavors in life that feel like too much.

Only joy, no pain

Throughout my athletic journey, I have experienced many different niggles, injuries, and obstacles. For a time, I used to experience nerve sensation in my feet during the run portion of a triathlon, typically a long course like half and full distances. At the time, I also made it a practice to have a session with MB during race week to talk about my mental strategy, mantra, and visualization. And so, this mantra came to life leading into the 2014 IRONMAN Lake Placid and was initially prescribed as simply the word "joy." MB said that if I were 100% focused on joy, I would be 0% focused on anything else. So during the marathon that day, I started reciting the mantra before the pain showed up, which was typically around mile eight, and when it did, I amended it to "only joy, no pain", which met my rhythm better and helped me stay focused to the finish line.

I'm not the doer

My first ultramarathon was the Mendocino 50K in 2017. It is best described in four words: river, ocean, redwoods, waterfall. With about four miles to go, the course turns into more of an obstacle course, complete with a 200-foot rope descent down a rocky cliff, strong winds along the headlands on a singletrack that is no wider than the length of a single foot, and a final stretch of deep sand to the finish. In the last two miles of my third running of this race in 2019, this mantra shouted itself through me. Quite literally, it came out of my mouth strong and loud. Although a part of me was saying, "you sound like a crazy person," I fully surrendered to the energy of these words and leaned into their power as chaos raged in my body. I was carried by something more powerful than I that day, and it helped me clock my fastest finish time.

Perfect steps

After running the Mendocino 50k in 2017 and having a superb experience, I went on the hunt for another ultra. The Black Mountain 50k was slated for June and was local to me in San Diego. I signed up. I heard rumblings about this ultra within the local trail community, most of which were unfavorable. Its technical landscape and reputation for heat were fertile ground for complaints. But there are a few, like me, who love this mountain. We find beauty in its gnarliness and respect the adversity it lends to its visitors. I have run this mountain countless times, and she has offered me stunning views from above the clouds, rapidly rising temperatures, quad-pounding descents, and epic face-first falls. I had a relationship with this mountain, and I thought I knew what I was getting into, but then again, you never really know what you're getting into, right?

Despite the rumblings, race day conditions were perfect; overcast through mile 15 of my race with Otter Pops[12] at the hottest part of the day atop the mountain's highest peak, which we hit at mile 25 of the race (nice touch, RD[13]). After the descent, the course took us back to a section lined with slick manzanita trees and offered some of the least technical trails. But then, to finish, we had to traverse some of the rockiest areas yet.

The sun was blasting, the temperature cranked, and with hot, dry conditions combined with the constant jostling from running, my sensitive eyes started to lose focus. I've experienced this before; it's when I hand over my experience to something greater and trust. The final three miles of this race were no different; my vision was compromised, and fatigue set in, but my competitive drive was 100%, pushing me harder and faster with each step. I caught up with a new friend of mine towards the end. It was his first ultra. He is a much faster runner than I am, but I had the honor to pull him home that day. He stayed

12 Otter Pops are a brand of freezies; frozen flavored ice pops.
13 RD is a commonly used acronym for Race Director who is the person who oversees, coordinates and implements a racing event.

on my heels, and we pushed in silence. I felt him struggling and hanging on to my strength in those moments. "Perfect steps," I told him, "that's the mantra; stay focused; let's go."

My vision continued to disintegrate, and the rocks were relentless, but the miles clicked off, and perfect steps took me home to a new personal best 50k finish time.

I am awake and ready

I crossed the finish line at the Cape Cod Marathon in 2009 and described it as the easiest marathon I've ever run. It was a great day; I ran a great marathon, got a great PR[14], and deemed it a great success. However, when I crossed that same finish line again in 2011, beating my previous time, it was after pushing through some of the most intense pain I have ever experienced.

I studied with Meditator Bob a few days before, and he gave me a new mantra to practice, "I am awake and ready." It resonated with me immediately, but after saying it a few times, I said, "Bob, I love it, but kind of think you're throwing me into the lion's den with this one." He laughed and did not waver on his recommendation. It felt like an invocation that was conjuring up something big. So, with this energy looming, what do you think I did?

Well, I distinctly recall saying outloud, "Bring it on, universe. You wanna dance, let's dance. I am awake and ready."

---

14 PR is an acronym for a personal record. It is widely used to describe an athlete's fastest time based on distance, pace, or course and can be in training or racing.

Race day arrived, and let's see, how about we start with the storm? I heard from one news outlet that we had not seen a storm like it since the Civil War. The temperature on race day was in the 30s with sky-high humidity and 60-70 mph wind gusts. Before leaving the car that day, my body was already chilled to the bone. If you know wet cold, then you know what I was experiencing.

I had recently recovered from a stress reaction in my tibia, which had me pool running and training at no more than 75% of my body weight on an anti-gravity treadmill leading into the marathon. So not only was my body not fully acclimated to running but the downed trees and branches strewn about the course served as additional obstacles.

Just curious, is there any force of nature that warrants a race cancellation in New England?

In gathering my gear from the car before heading to the starting line, I realized I needed more fuel, and although the race guide said there would be gels at the aid stations, I was informed that morning there were none. I had what I had, salt capsules, three gels, six glucose tabs, a boatload of will, and my mantra. I needed all of it, the mantra, the fuel, and the faith and belief in something greater than me.

That day, I learned that I was tough, New England tough, but mostly, that I can persevere as long as "I am awake and ready." It would be years until I learned the art of ease and the peace of equanimity, but on this day, I danced with the power of the universe and, if my memory serves me, ran a personal best marathon time.

Om namah shivaya

MB once told me that the challenges get bigger and the path becomes narrow as we evolve. And this makes sense if you look at what our modern world promotes and celebrates. It is not the 10,000-foot view or truths of self-realization that sell to the masses; it's good news about bad habits and quick-fix hacks that sell best. He also taught me that solitude is the price of success. By the time I heard this, I had learned that I am not alone even when alone, which is often, so this did not scare me. If all life emerges from the same essence, then we are never alone because we are connected by that essence which is the lifeline that unites us all. As our commitment to sit becomes non-negotiable, we become more familiar with that essence and we trust more. Trust allows us to lean into surrender, which is what this mantra is about—om namah shivaya, "I surrender to the divine."

As a spectator and race participant, I have relied on this mantra countless times, for example, on multiple occasions when BJ has been carried into the medical tent after crossing a finish line. And in many moments when I bore the weight of the world, like when our first golden retriever Harry was getting ready to transition from his body, and there was nothing I could do to ease his suffering. I have used this mantra to increase my trust and in times when I needed to pick myself up from the rubble of sadness. Not many days pass, especially as an entrepreneur and awake athlete on the path to mastery, when I do not relax into its translation. And I do not foresee a time when I will deny the power or beauty I feel when I merge with our divine universe and surrender into its arms.

AUM (OM)

All of the mantras previously mentioned and otherwise, culminate into one vibration. Every vibration equals this one vibration; every crying baby, every laughing being, the shrill of a scream, and carefulness of a whisper. Every animal roaring and cawing, every dumpster being opened and slammed closed, and every wave breaking on the shore—all of it. Every sound, when united, creates the eternal vibration of one, aum.

Aum articulates in three audible sounds followed by silence. *Ahhhh* represents the waking state or the beginning. *Uhhhh* represents the dream state or the middle, the sustenance of life as we know it. *Mmmmm* represents the deep sleep state or the beginning of the end. And then silence which represents absolute consciousness, being one with Self.

Although I knew about this mantra for decades, I had never used it during a racing event until November 29, 2015 when BJ and I celebrated our 13th wedding anniversary by competing at IRONMAN Cozumel. In our session before I left for Mexico, MB told me to drop all mantras and only use aum for this race. Despite resistance from the mind telling me it was too simple, I took his guidance. I feared it wouldn't be enough, but I knew far too well that I needed to do it if MB said. I had enough skin in the game to allow but not indulge the voice of doubt, so I took my spiritual strategy across the border.

A few yards into the swim, I felt the jellyfish sting my leg, then my hand, then my face, *Ah-Uh-Mm.*

When the wind blew like it was the end of days on the island's east side, *Ah-Uh-Mm.*

When a house fire on the course had me riding my bike through a cloud of thick black smoke, *Ah-Uh-Mm,* and when a blister broke open during the run and the unprotected nerves rubbed against my sock, *Ah-Uh-Mm.*

In the chaos of swimming 2.4 miles, biking 112 miles, and running 26.2 miles in hot, windy conditions, *Ah-Uh-Mm* and another PR.

GUIDED MEDITATION

Utilizing the tools of breath and mantra to concentrate the mind is all you need to reach the higher levels of consciousness where all things are possible (ahem, PR heaven on earth). But what about guided meditations? I get this question regularly.

They are fabulous; they are one of my favorite tools to create and provide for athletes. I practice them regularly. But not as my primary practice. I reserve my morning practice for my higher Self and me only. I use guided meditations during my second practice but not all the time. I know MB would prefer I ditch them entirely because guided meditations are guidance that comes from outside of us. He taught me that they can be helpful and will get you on base, but they won't get you to home plate. You want the guidance of a teacher along this path, but when it comes to your daily meditation, taking the direct route inward is considered best. You cannot be wholly focused inward when you partially focus on the external. In this case, the meditation teacher guiding you through the practice.

Guided meditations are like cold-pressed juice sold off the shelf of a grocery store. These juices undergo a pasteurization process to sustain shelf-life, dulling the nutrition's vibrancy. The alternative is to go to an organic juice bar that uses a slow masticating juicer, does not pasteurize, and provides you with the biggest bang of nutrition that only fresh, organic, cold-pressed juice delivers. Now, if all you can get is juice from a grocery store, then, by all means, proceed because it will benefit you. But if you have a juice bar around the corner with integrity and are able to pay for the highest vibration, I will choose that for you every time.

WAKE. PEE. MEDITATE.
There is no better recipe than this recipe for committing to sit. I know this because it's the one I've used since day one, as prescribed by my teacher and many other teachers throughout the ages. I now prescribe it for you.

At the start of my meditation journey, I recognized that I was not trustworthy to push my meditation to later in the day. Wake, pee, meditate allowed me to counteract the voice that tried to convince me that later was better. It told me that I would feel better and the meditation would be more profound if I just got a few things done or off my mind first, but time and again, that reality failed to come to fruition. Any voice that tells you that you don't have time or it will be better later because you need to get things done first is telling you lies.

I know that not all of you are early morning people, but I highly encourage the shift because the early morning hours between 4 am and 6 am are genuinely sacred times to meditate. Our physical surroundings are quiet, daily distractions are at an all-time low, and there is less pressure to be doing. In addition, the day's momentum has not yet begun to stir, and it is the ideal time to consciously create momentum for your day.

Because your mind and body are not active yet, deeper states of meditation are more accessible. If your body feels stiff or uncomfortable, it's helpful to perform a few yoga poses such as cat/cow, down dog, and sun salutations to promote circulation and flexibility of the body. The asanas or postures of yoga are meant for this very thing, to prepare the body for stillness.

Regarding where you should meditate, do not underestimate your closet, bathroom, or space on the floor next to your bed as a private ashram. I've worked with many athletes entertaining rationalizations about their inability to meditate because of their family or lack of dedicated space. They cannot wake their husband or kids by walking down the creaky stairs. I have heard and experienced the many obstacles to meditation, but remember, there are limitless solutions to every problem. We just need to be willing to step into the new world mind of solution energy.

Athletes who go beyond the excuses of the small self find great solace in closets and bathrooms as places to fulfill their wake, pee, meditate pledge. Bonuses no one saw coming include keeping these spaces cleaner than before. Decluttering the mind also comes with decluttering all things in life, material and otherwise. A nudge back to Tashi's perspective-shifting clutter comment, as we attune to the clutterless part of us, we will also realize that in our outer world.

If you have thoughts on why you cannot wake, pee, and meditate, then I challenge you to challenge each of those so-called reasons by taking cues from Byron Katie's life-changing work, *The Work*, and ask yourself:

1) Is this thought true?

2) How do you know it's true if the answer is yes?

3) Then ask yourself, is there a stress-free reason to keep the thought or belief?

I challenge you to prove the time-tested wake, pee, meditate recipe for entering each day from a state of unitive presence is flawed or wrong. Go ahead, be an experiment of one and show yourself the truth.

A RECIPE FOR SITTING

This chapter contains everything you need to tame your mind, elevate your life and become the powerful creator you came here to be. But I know it's still not enough for the part of the mind that always needs more. I mean, there's no way that breathing, mantra, and stillness every day will change everything, let alone anything, without a concrete set of steps. So, let's gather the ingredients and put the recipe together.

If this is day one of meditation for you, start simple and keep it simple for the rest of your life. If you are returning to your practice like you do every day, let this be a reminder to keep it simple for the rest of your life. Ready? Here we go:

1) Take a comfortable seat with your back straight. You can sit in a chair, against a wall with a pillow supporting your back, or on a cushion. The key is to be comfortable. If we are comfortable, we create a safe relationship with meditation, and it will be easier to return. It is essential to find the sweet spot between ease and effort just like your "all day pace" in training. Be patient because meditative posture is physical training, but with consistency and curiosity, your body will find the sweet spot.

2) Set a meditation timer for 10-20 minutes (or longer if you are a regular meditator) but it also works if you only have five minutes. Just like physical training, consistency is everything.

3) Close your eyes and bring your awareness to your breath. This is not about stopping your thoughts. It's a practice of deliberate focus.

4) Use three of the pranayama exercises. If you can't choose, allow me: three-part breath, tense and release, and relaxing breath. Complete each breath exercise one time if meditating

for 10 minutes and three times if meditating for 20 minutes or longer.

5) After your final breath exercise, release control of the breath and take a moment to notice how you feel without indulging in the commentary about how you feel.

6) Begin the mantra "so hum". Think *soooo* on the inhale and *hummm* on the exhale. Remember, this vibration manifests as peace. Feel the words instead of just thinking and linking them together. Meditation is not a task to tick off your list. It is a deep feeling, slowing down encounter with the present moment.

7) You will return to your thought-life at some point, okay, many points, throughout your meditation, especially at first. When you find yourself there, refocus your attention on the mantra. If you get frustrated, remind yourself that your busy mind doesn't make you a less than meditator, and it never warrants an abandonment of the practice.

8) When you feel calm, release the mantra, bring awareness to your heart or the center of your forehead above your eyebrows and rest deeply in silence.

During this part I sometimes rest my attention on my heart, I focus on feeling that space and imagining the energy of love. I let it expand with every breath, I fill my home and the beings in my house with that love, and then I share it with my neighbors. Eventually, I wrap the entire globe in that love, as envisioned as white light, and then I pull my focus out and see our earth; the oceans, the animals, the humans, and all of nature surrounded and absorbed with this love. I rest here.

Other times I focus on my third eye, the center of my forehead, and imagine a long tunnel with a bright white light at the end of that tunnel. I envision myself walking down the tunnel and stepping into the light. This vision typically morphs into watching the entire universe, its galaxies and constellations. I rest here.

This recipe is the blueprint that I started with and practice to this day with a few variations. I include a chakra clearing, alternate nostril breathing, and more beingness at the end. After a time, it is common to have an athlete tell me they are bored with their meditation and need a change. However, these are not reasons to change the practice; this boredom is the mind demanding entertainment. And the more we feed its unceasing need to be distracted, the more difficult it will be to tame it down the line.

So what do you do with a demanding mind? Let it exhaust itself naturally, and be sure to breathe consciously throughout its antics. Your attention is the invitation. As we engage with thoughts, we give them fuel. Like a child having a tantrum, allow it to run its course. Let the demands come and go. Eventually, the mind will quiet down and allow you to go deep.

As you build your practice, increase the length of your daily meditation or incorporate one extended meditation per week. The increased time gives the mind space to tantrum and surrender while you get better at allowing it all to come and go. As the surface interference of the mind dissipates, we enter deeper states of presence which is the only place we can learn about deeper states of presence. Meditation has been shown to slow down the brain's default mode network activity, which is a part of the brain implicated in mind wandering. So yes, there is more quiet coming into your practice and life. Continue without attachment to the timeline, and your mind will grow tame to your command.

When it came to Clark, we had two choices; invest time and money to train him or let him run amuck. The latter was not an option. Of course it was not an option; anyone would agree. So if this is true about our pups, why is it not true about our minds?

With the mind at the helm, our realities are created haphazardly and by default. Some things work out, and some things do not. Some days are good, and some days are bad. Some days, the puppy chews on the furniture; some days, we get off easy. For too long, we have been pulled around by our mind-stuff, like a dog on a leash. Please do not be fooled by this misplaced master any longer. Through a daily practice of observance and choices, redirects, and non-resistance, you send a continuous stream of messaging to the mind that you are the one holding the end of the leash. And just like every well-behaved pup, it will soon enough realize that service is where it thrives.

CHAPTER SEVEN

POWER OF THE PAUSE

"This is a pathless path. Where the journey leads is to the deepest truth in you. It is really just returning to where you were before you got lost."

Ram Dass

I completed my first yoga teacher training in 2013 with Live, Love, Teach (LLT), a groundbreaking yoga teacher training program dedicated to turning out exceptional instructors. Teachers who are redefining modern-day marketable yoga. LLT founder Philip Urso ran the training I attended. I have mentioned him a time or two already in this book.

I met Philip on my 39th birthday when I attended his class at Inner Light Yoga in Middletown, RI. I knew within the first words he spoke that he was my teacher. There was an authenticity about him that was incredibly easeful and believable. He was passionate, open-hearted, and dropped the "F" bomb in class, which was the ultimate cool for me.

Although Philip often said over the years that he wouldn't have to swear if he was more intelligent. He said it was lazy. And it is. I agree now, but at that time, all I wanted to do was drop an "F" bomb in a yoga class, and I knew he could teach me how.

Before breaking out on his own, Philip studied with world-renowned yogi Baron Baptiste for many years. He resonated with the power vinyasa model of controlling the breath to move from pose to pose. When practiced earnestly, this form of breath and flow becomes a deeply connected, moving meditation—like the pouring oil pranayama technique from chapter six, absolutely seamless. Philip was discovering the power of breath-focused vinyasa, and his curiosity drove him to learn more about being an effective yoga teacher. Over time through his experience, he grew curious about the effect that more silence, increased focus on the breath, and the removal of music could have on a practitioner's experience. So he took the learned principles and experimented with how far he could take them. He found what I and many others have also found; when we strip away distractions, we become familiar with the timelessness of the present moment, and this is where we access the pauses of life. These pauses are the space between stimulus and response, and they are all over the place in your life.

Class after class, whether teaching or practicing, I noticed that just like there are peaks and valleys everywhere in life, there are just as many moments to pause. And in the pause, everything slowed down, including me. I never experienced anything like this before in my life. It was a blatant sign that yoga was teaching me something completely new and I was ready for it. I felt so comforted by where I was at that time in my life. I remember such sure-footedness about being in those classes, that training, and then stepping up as an instructor. My dharma was becoming clear, and the feeling matched what I had long felt in my core.

Following India, becoming a yoga instructor was my next big awakening. A large part of this awakening was learning about the ego. An education that began on the first day of training when Philip had us get up in front of everyone and teach. If you ever want to see your ego, instruct a room full of people you do not know, including a handful of well-versed yoga instructors, to sweep their arms up and breathe in. It may sound easy, but it was certifiably painful. I wanted to be the best at it, and I felt internal pressure to be better than all the rest, which resulted in one of my worst performances yet.

Looking back now, though, it was one of my most valuable training experiences. I hear many stories of teachers coming out of their 200-hour teacher training with little to no teaching time. They then find themselves standing in front of a class with a lot of information about poses and philosophy but minimal experience guiding students into situations where they can actually practice yoga. I have also heard stories about memorized scripts for teaching and instructors who can only teach by practicing as they teach. These feel like heavy ways to teach a yoga class. LLT not only had us teaching on the first day and every day throughout the training, but we also gained the experience of leading a public class before graduation.

Over the years, Philip identified a staggering absence of silence in yoga studios. He became adamant about doing away with the "wall of words" most often experienced in a yoga class. And so, in keeping with the commitment to limit external stimuli in the classroom, we received consistent instruction throughout our training to talk as little as possible. By using minimum relevant words throughout a class, I can focus more on observing the class. Then through what I observe, I can discern what the class needs, if anything. For example, if I say, "left foot forward, warrior one," and see most students struggling to figure it out, I will offer a queue. If it is just a few students, I will give them more space, allow them to look around, and try to find it in their bodies. And in my experience, the vast majority of the time, the correct answer is always more silence and space.

Silence is not easy at first, especially since it is uncommon in yoga classes and largely in our society. Still, by skillfully reminding students of perfect tools like breath awareness, they learn to navigate silence and the mental noise that may arise within it. The breath keeps us concentrated on the moment where the pause exists. This pause is where we can choose a new direction for our mind and override patterns that no longer serve us, like the discomfort pattern we have become accustomed to in silence because of all distractions in life.

The pause, although difficult to see at first, is magical because it is where change occurs. One of our biggest obstacles to change is that we live in bodies hardwired for survival and energy conservation. It's the part of us that says change does not need to occur because changing the known leads to the unknown, which feels too risky. It reasons that walking into the unknown is more threatening than the misery of staying the same. Therefore, the mind will automatically choose the known over the unknown, even if it causes pain and suffering.

This is why we see people keep themselves from joy, remain in professions they loathe, and stay away from what they truly desire. As Diane Collins describes in her book, *Do You Quantum Think?* it is the myth of choice. We think we are always making choices, but in reality, our choices are being made by our patterns. Many of these automatic cycles are helpful to living in the world, for example, stopping at red lights and good oral hygiene, but many are keeping us distanced from our true nature. Those are the ones we want to be conscious around, and that requires us to get really comfy in the pause.

For me, there was no pause for many years, okay, decades. Like many of you, I lived under the myth of choice for most of my life, but yoga was waking me up in my late thirties, and I had the determination to change because, as clear as day, I could see my misery. I knew I had to override the patterns keeping me the same and venture into the unknown version of me if I wanted to be happy. Yoga gave me the tools to be successful, and I felt a volume of momentum that was effortlessly drawing me closer to the authenticity I saw in Philip. I wanted more of it, and I kept hearing that it was in the present moment. So I practiced presence everywhere, as much as I could, and I continue to do so to this day. I am very much in the practice and the authenticity that I now live within continues to expand with each moment.

As an instructor, I constantly monitor the voice in my head that pressures me to say something spiritual or tries to tell me that the class I'm teaching isn't enough. It means I practice teaching in a way that is not about my small self but in a manner that serves the community as a whole, of which I am a part. As I watch my own impulses and automatic responses, I am teaching the students to do the same. My job for them is to hold the space, drop in the tools, and watch the class. By giving students simple tools like putting 100% of their awareness on their breath, they begin to learn, just as I did, that there is a space between the commentary and where their awareness resides. When we focus on something other than our thoughts, we witness the tendencies of our minds. As we do this, we can deliberately steer ourselves through life with conscious awareness to a position of true power.

Yoga is the science of the mind, after all, and although it is helpful to assist a student who is creating an unhelpful pattern in their body, I have seen very few lives change on account of the angle of a foot within a pose. Suppose someone knocks your bike over in the transition area at a triathlon just as you finish stacking it with nutrition and resting your helmet and sunglasses perfectly on the bars. At that moment, it will not matter if you can perform a perfectly aligned warrior pose. What makes the difference is if you can get into the pause, take a conscious breath to interrupt thoughts that you are a victim, and respond from your 10,000-foot view big neutral Self. This does not mean that you cannot or will not have emotions. You are going to have feelings. Stuff is going ignite anger and fear for the rest of the time you are on this earth. If life promises anything, it's that we will experience a full range of emotions along our paths.

In my growth in this area, learning the truth about emotions was helpful because I was feeling so much in the pause and it felt overwhelming at times. I learned that emotions are simply *energy in motion*. From the 10,000-foot view, the person who knocked your bike over is actually in service of you. They are the guru, the catalyst for that *energy in motion* to rise up while the pause allows you to no longer create from it. Our focus is the invitation. So, if we focus on anger, we expand anger. If we focus on calm, we expand calm. As we focus on our thoughts, we will have more thoughts. If we focus on the quiet within, we will experience more quiet from within.

At first, there will only be glimpses, but over time, a little bit every day, you will recondition the mind, repattern the brain, and improve your life and performance. As we get more familiar with the pause, we see people, experiences, and emotions in their truth. And there is only one truth; it's love. Love is a neutral space where we can break historical patterns and heal ancestral karma active in our DNA and soul body. To wake up to the energy of love is to learn that each moment is a moment to begin again and that instant forgiveness allows us to exceed far beyond what we are conditioned to believe is possible. There was, you know, a time before all the conditioning, and it was right at the start of our lives, the time when everything was perfect.

With a perfect energy match between our soul and our parent's souls, our earthly life begins as we drop into the physical body of our mother. While in the womb, we trust everything that happens; we live in the pause of the present moment. We are not yet conditioned to be fearful or anxious about *what is*. Dr. Wayne Dyer, spiritual author no longer on this earth, often discussed this phase of life when we are non-resistant to our development.

As our noses grow, we do not complain. We do not worry as our lungs form and we know we are enough as our brains evolve. Then about ten earth months into our flow of life, we journey down the amnesia portal, known as the birth canal, and into the world of conditions where we are categorized within the modem of modern life. We begin moving away from our inner being by turning our focus to the outer world, one that dismisses the eternal wisdom we hold within.

We learn that we must achieve to get ahead, and getting ahead is imperative because if we are not ahead, we must be behind. This earth is a dualistic world that denies our non-dualistic nature, and because of this, we get lost. The survival of the fittest mentality is baked into our minds, and it is a terrifying way to live; one that has driven us to a society of safetyism[15]. We are so busy being fearful of fear that we completely forget who we are and we get lost.

15 The concept of *safetyism* is defined and discussed by authors, Greg Lukianoff and Jonathan Haidt in their book *The Coddling of the American Mind*. It is a cultural belief system that expands the concept of safety beyond physical and into the emotional. It's a mindset that intends to protect but may actually be increasing our fragility as humans and denying our nature as resilient creatures.

I got lost. You got lost. And it is this disconnection from our truth that enhances frustration, fear, anxiety, and other emotions that keep us from greatness. I am not immune to life's challenges and the colorful flavor of *energy in motion*. This book, in its entirety, is the ethos of my awakening, and there were many years of me living lost and without pause. It was not until I stepped onto the yoga mat that it all blew up in my face.

It was the early 1990s in Newport, at the old Waterfront Fitness, a small gym on the second floor of a historic downtown building along famed America's Cup Avenue. I walked into the aerobics room, which we called it back then, and rolled out a yoga mat for the second time in my life. And although no one forced me into that room that day, I begrudgingly reached my fingers to the sky, felt mother earth under my feet, and thought much of what I was hearing was nonsense. Then, approximately a quarter of the way through class, the instructor guided us into warrior II and told us to hold the pose.

I estimate it was no longer than 20 seconds before I glared at the instructor with a gaze hot enough to bore holes into her skull. I entertained visions of yelling at her from my mat and accidentally harming her while making a dramatic exit as a volcanic eruption arose from within. An unrelenting voice screamed that I get out of the pose. Instead, I stayed.

My mind hurled into a stream of victimizing thoughts while a burning inferno of intolerable sensation showed me my lack of strength. Anger flared, but I refused to be defeated by a stagnate hold. I was more powerful than yoga, and I would not give up. I endured the pose and the rest of the class, including savasana, which felt like a colossal waste of time. I decided at least ten times that yoga and I were done forever. But, just like the race you swear you will never race again, I found myself on the mat just a few days later.

More than three decades later, I find my way to the mat as often as possible. Over the years, I've discovered more protection and peace on that rectangle than anywhere else. I love warrior II, and savasana is my favorite pose. I've come a long way from wanting to harm the teacher, and as I gaze upon it now, I see that instructor planted the first seeds in my education of the pause.

When I look back on that yoga class, I see a girl overloaded with egoic impulses and acting on those without inquiry into their validity. I see a girl who used her will to push and manipulate situations. I see a girl who would flow in and out of her center many times a day. A girl who had strong intuition but had not yet truly begun to awaken. It would be another fifteen years before I walked into Philip's class and when I did I finally felt like I was coming home. I had spent so many years running from myself but that day, I turned around.

Under his guidance, I practiced watching my breath and not responding to every mental impulse in class. I worked with MB regularly and sat in meditation each morning to concentrate my mind. It was a battle royale. I also began to study the Gita. I was deep in the battle of the mind and learning about where my mind was dwelling. I kept paying close attention to what I was doing while I was doing it, and as a result, I deepened my relationship with the present moment. From here, I began to experience an effortless shift in awareness where being present became easier.

Being present opened space for me to see how I moved through my days—a phase I call *getting onto yourself*. It's when we see what we can no longer unsee. It is the point of no return. I heard my annoying comebacks and moments when I fought for my limitations with increasing volume. I started to feel the judgment, lack, and jealousy in my experiences and realized that the perceived power from which I believed I was responding was nothing but a one-way ticket to nowhere. I saw cycles repeat daily and decided to no longer stay the same. At first, the pause was brief, but even a glance left me wanting more. With more practice, I learned to hang in the pause at my leisure while allowing a thought or impulse to pass through without engaging with it. Each time I let it be there without fueling it, my ability to remain breath-aware grew stronger, and the effects translated into my everyday life.

Yoga helped me slow the speed of the internal tornado of my thought-life; I felt the layers loosen and more room in my life overall. I felt it everywhere; in my cycles with BJ, my food choices, my alcohol choices, and my word choices. More, more, more. I just wanted more. This is what the awakening spark will do. It will open you to a power that may be unknown to you and to its fullest extent, is unknown to me. Yet, even one instant in the pause grants you access to the inner calm that is your invincible essence of mastery.

A breathing technique that deepens familiarity with the pause is to linger in the space between breaths. Try it, even for an instant, at the top of the inhale and bottom of the exhale. As you get more familiar, wait until the impulse to breathe arises, then wait for another few heartbeats before welcoming the breath. This technique provides the physical benefits of stretching and strengthening the lungs and accessory breathing muscles which sharpens the awake athlete edge and reinforces the power of pausing before we take a new direction.

The pause allows for mastery when you are killing it on the downhill of an ultramarathon and realize you are off course and the only way back is to climb the trail you just descended. It's also in those times when you finally feel ahead in your finances and receive a bill for an overdue medical procedure that your insurance company said they would pay many months ago. The pause is a moment in time when you are free to choose. Free to respond. Free to release feelings of victimhood and transcend the voice of the ego so that you may live the demonstration of what you desire to see more of in the world. And it's all yours for the choosing.

Choose if you will be a crappy runner or the runner you've always dreamed of becoming. Choose if you are going to let outside circumstances determine your mood. Choose if you will fight or surrender to the state of what is. Choose if you will hand your power over to your life circumstance and become powerless in your chosen victimhood. For it is only within a moment of witnessing that we get to make another choice, so we best pay attention because the life we desire and the athlete we strive to be is always one choice away. And that choice lives right now in the powerful pause.

CHAPTER EIGHT

EGO IS NOT YOUR ENEMY

"The momentum towards unification in oneness with all creation is underway. The force of that momentum is a fact of life itself and cannot be impeded for the power of love is quite literally unstoppable."

Rasha

Over the past few decades of working within varying healing arts professions, I have heard many excuses. I am well-versed in why people can't stretch, why they can't do yoga, and always why they can't meditate. When I see mouths open and words start to come, I swear I'm open to hearing something valid, but alas, I have yet to hear anything but excuses.

I wrote this first paragraph several years ago, and it helps to hear it with a tone of overconfidence that was common for me back then. I mean, I knew a lot about living a good life. I was well-educated on the physical body and thriving as a massage therapist and yoga instructor. My intention was always to leave people feeling better than when they arrived, and I knew I was blessed to play such a role in life. But people relied on my guidance in the yoga studio and my skills in tissue manipulation, and I allowed that reliance to exist and expand. I did not know any better at the time. I liked being the source of healing for others and believed I held their answers. I did not see the truth that their answers lived inside them. If I'm to be fully honest, there were times I held back in fear that they would no longer need me if I told them everything.

And although there is nothing wrong with job satisfaction, I often asserted my worth on how much people needed me and how they did or did not heal, and that was problematic. When they didn't recover or didn't return to class or my treatment room, I condemned either myself for not being good enough or them for not doing the work. When I saw students that attended my class show up in other teachers' classes, I felt threatened and unworthy. And so, although I intended to assist others in living a better life and, by all means, people were living better lives under my guidance, something was getting in the way that kept me from a pure heart, a humble heart which I now know is a powerful heart. But back then, I didn't want much to do with a humble heart; a strong force said I held the keys to the kingdom, and it was bound and determined to hand out copies as it readily saw fit.

I feel constriction and a lack of compassion in the first paragraph of this chapter, and I now understand the words I wrote have more to do with me than anyone else. I see that I felt invalid, and I projected those feelings onto the reasonings of others. I allowed my perspective to come through the narrow viewfinder of my ego, which led to compulsive feelings of trumped-up worthiness, detrimental unworthiness, and blame of self or another.

Over the years, my heart has opened. It has been a slow process helped tremendously by looking up compassion in the dictionary, even if it was a lot to swallow at first. I had heard the term but didn't know what it meant. I remember reading something along the lines of feeling another's suffering as my own, and I cringed. Nevertheless, it was a good reference point for where I was on my path to an open heart because that was the last thing I wanted to do. Their suffering was on them, not me. I had enough on my plate. I wasn't going to start taking on the suffering of others. Absolutely not; I'll take a pass.

MB identified intolerance, compassion's opposite, as an early theme with me. As he and my study with LLT guided me to look within, not surprisingly, I found self-intolerance at the root. It has taken time and will continue to take time. The soul's evolution is a process spiritual leader Ram Dass described as painfully slow, but as the student is ready and clutter falls away, it does so effortlessly. All we have to do is stay the course.

Through this long, slow process, I have awakened to patience, and it never pressures, judges, or punishes me for anything. Instead, it rests in an inherent trust that all is in right order while not excusing me from repaying the debts of my actions. I have become more acquainted with this energy through time and practice, which has changed me on a cellular level. I hear it in my tone, experience it in my health, and read it in my words. And these shifts prove true for all who walk the path of awakening.

As clutter continues to fall, I notice more ease around previously challenging things, like listening to excuses. I hear the truth in every word, and I better relate to the athlete because I can see myself in them. As we open to self-acceptance, we naturally extend acceptance to all. This energy is that of the true Self, and as we get to know that part of ourselves better, we notice the false self, more commonly known as the ego.

In one class with Philip, who studied *A Course in Miracles*[16], I learned that every loving thought is true; everything else is a cry for help and healing, no matter the form it takes. This was another Tashi at the cafe moment because, from then on, I questioned non-loving thoughts. And as I turned inward to look where those non-loving thoughts were coming from, I saw a part of me crying for help and healing—the less-than part of me, the voice that cried victim and often placed blame.

I had learned a lot already about free will, you know, from lingering in the powerful pause, so I decided to use it to

---

16 *A Course In Miracles*, also known as ACIM or simply the Course, is a self-study guide that when practiced leads us to the recognition of love in all things. From the acim.org website, "A Course In Miracles (ACIM) is a unique spiritual self-study program designed to awaken us to the truth of our oneness with God and Love". There is no author attributed to this work as it was scribed through Dr. Helen Schucman, a clinical and research psychologist. She asserts that over the course of seven years, from 1965 - 1972, the Course was received via inner dictation; word by word from Jesus Christ. It all began with the following directive, "This is a course in miracles, please take notes."

entertain new perspectives in attempt to heal my sub-par way of being. This was when my inward journey started to pay dividends, making me long for more. I looked to where I was offering excuses instead of pursuing my greatness. After the initial shock of finding what I found unacceptable in others within me, I saw that every one of my excuses held true for me. The excuse reflected where I was, and instead of working forward from a place of acceptance, I had been choosing self-unacceptance and projecting my frustration onto others doing the same.

As my awareness grew, my ability to allow things to be as they are also increased, making it easier to steer my thoughts back into alignment since I wasn't fighting the present moment so much. As I accepted myself, intolerance faded into understanding. And with understanding, I found patience. In patience, I learned to trust, and with the expansion of this greater part of myself, I saw the power I was handing over to the ego. And although this path required me to feel the intense pain I had suppressed, all of the changes I realized were effortless, as Ram Dass described. I was getting to know myself well, and it became the solution for everything that ailed me.

I was seeing the false self for the first time with new eyes. I saw myself in the eyes of others and felt their pain as my own. And although the ego has not gone away, it has shifted from its previously solely small and limiting reality to assisting me in making the positive changes I desire. My ego is becoming my teammate because it understands its position within the hierarchy of me. This understanding does not mean the battle of the mind is over, but I am getting better at playing the game. Better and better, every day in every way.

Most of us live in ego-identification. We see, taste, feel, hear, and smell life experiences through the narrow viewfinder of the false self. It's the primary mode from which most live because we are seen as separate, and it keeps us from the expansive life we came here to experience and the gifts we hold a responsibility to share.

We embody separation in our languaging, actions, and beliefs. My family, your family. Nature, human, animal. My gender, your gender, genderless. Anti-vax, pro-vax, meditator, manic. Our identification with the ego and the idea that we are separate accounts for every problem in our life experiences. We are unique, that is true and critical to the fabric of humanity, but we are not independent of one another. There is a common denominator, and some call it God, Universe, Source, Science, Mother Nature, Allah, or Jesus. Regardless of the label, the essence of all is exact, and we are individualized reflections of this source. All titles are merely a label that allows us to feel the God of our unique understanding in a way that we are ready to embody. Here's a way of visualizing what I just stated, which helped me tremendously in my learning; I hope it does the same for you:

Imagine a row of buckets on a bright sunny day. They are lined up next to one another and filled with water. Life is the bucket, we are the water, and the sun is our source. When you look into each bucket, you see the sun's reflection, but because the buckets sit within their unique space, the sun's reflection on the water is slightly different for each. Yet, regardless of their unique position, the sun shines on all buckets and water with the same intensity. It does not block its rays from any of them. Clouds float in front of this light all the time, which makes it harder to see, but the light never ceases to shine. In the Gita, Krishna tells Arjuna that he holds the entire cosmos with only a fragment of his being. We are reflections of that being. And although it is in us, we are not in it.

There is something greater out there keeping it all together, and it is what connects us all, loves us all, and accepts us all in our uniqueness. I have found great wonder and daily reverence in acknowledging that the universe is still holding together when my alarm goes off each morning. And as Michael Singer suggests in *The Untethered Soul*, I often zoom out to remember that I am a speck on a gigantic ball spinning in the middle of nowhere. Simple yet expansive practices like these assist us in residing within the 10,000-foot view of life. They helps us hold the bigger picture so we can steer ourselves toward life's solutions and re-discover our truth.

The ego has a tough time seeing the big picture because it solely identifies with its perception of the natural world. It carries a false sense of power (ahem, overconfident tone) and a denial that there is one plan, timeline, and dream—the dream of God. Compassion was my catalyst to learn about the ego and the same tool I have found crucial in guiding the ego. We don't want to punish the ego because punishment is egoic energy. Therefore, we must guide ourselves from a connection with our truest nature of love and allow the ego to become a beloved tool in our toolbox.

One evening during yoga training, I asked how to define the ego, and Philip told me that the ego is a separation device. Me from you, they from them, and this from that. "Okay," I thought, "so the opposite of connection." My curiosity around this drove me to pay particular attention to when I felt disconnected, which ended up feeling the same way as when I noticed non-loving thoughts, which led to the realization that the man behind the curtain is always the same (no offense, guys). And, we are either moving from connection with source or identification with ego.

I later learned from MB that ego energy carries our free will, a significant component of driving ourselves to reach a goal. The ego represents our individuality, and we need this as citizens of the earth. This planet is an ego world. If it were not an ego world, there would be no war, race, gluttony, starvation, night, or day. It's a land of contrast, and it serves a particular purpose. We are not made for this world; this world is made for us, and so our collective goal as awake athletes is to learn how this world works because mastery is very much about mastering our existence in the physical realm.

As it is now, for most of you, the ego is not your teammate and frequently works against you, not because it is your enemy but because you were never taught to be the master of it. The yogis teach us the ego sits at the base of the skull in the medulla oblongata, the lowest part of the brain and the lowest portion of the brainstem. It situates on the same pole as the third eye chakra, the eye of wisdom, in the center of the forehead above the eyebrows. Living from the ego-eye view is like heading out on the trail at night with your headlamp on backward. It is how the masses live and the state of affairs that our society has gathered around for ages. The perpetual separateness of the ego means that it needs to be seen as a separate autonomous being. It manifests in many ways: the victim and the victimizer, winner, and loser, the one that is better than and the one that is less than. This voice constantly compares, pulling us up and down life's extremes while almost always wishing for another now. And even when it is satisfied, it's not for long.

The ego is the part of us that is excited to go on vacation and, once on vacation, thinks about how nice it will be to get home and back into a routine. It's the voice that signs up for an event that we have always wanted to do and then complains about the weather on race day. It's the part that chooses to dine outside and then wants to be inside and the part that wants so badly to get married and then feels trapped.

The ego shines outward from its singular view, and although it is not separate from our soul, it is, quite literally, our soul turned in the opposite direction. It is thoroughly identified with the physical world and believes three-dimensional old world living is all there is to know. In comparison, our eye of wisdom shines its new worldview from the penthouse perspective. It sees all the paths, solutions, and, no matter what needs to be traversed to get there, the grandest of all resolutions. As our relationship with Self deepens through the practice of meditation, the ego begins to turn and merge in with our wisdom eye. This is when the ego becomes our teammate, and we can start having much more joy in life, especially when setting and attaining goals. The key is to gently but firmly guide the ego. MB says, "relentless pressure consistently applied."

Athletes, don't fret. As of yet, waking up has not diminished my competitiveness. I love being competitive, and I love being competitive with myself, but that's not the whole truth, not even close. I love being competitive with others. This is where the ego assists me greatly. The reality is we are competing. There is a winner, and there is a loser. There is first over the line and last over the line. Since the ego thrives within separateness, competition is an excellent place for it to thrive, and as long as it is under our control, we can use its drive to our advantage.

Without our deliberate guidance, the ego will always make decisions from fear of the unknown and use history as a critical element in its decision-making process. This especially rings true when it comes to reaching new levels of success in any aspect of our life because anytime we go to better ourselves, we experience egoic resistance. Steven Pressfield wrote a fantastic book called the *War Of Art*. It's a short read focused on the energy of resistance that holds us back from success and one that helped me put knowledge into action during my pre-meditation days.

The ego's fear of change fuels repetitive cycles in our life, good and bad. Getting your meditation practice to be a least-action pathway in your life is good. Crowding out animal products on your plate with vibrant plant foods is good. Being more compassionate, honest, steadfast, and calm are good behaviors to store in your locked and loaded response locker.

However, patterns like regular disappointment are harmful. They do not lean you into excellence. Fear of getting injured or rained on during the race or hit by a car is bad. They are not helpful for your desire to feel peaceful and powerful. And although I label them as good and bad, no person is better than or less than for exhibiting any of these behaviors in their life, good or bad. The purpose of good is to confirm that we're on track and aligned. The purpose of bad is to show us what we don't want and that we have distanced ourselves from our center. By using this information to our advantage, we lead ourselves in the direction we desire. On the awake athlete path, use all experiences to align yourself with your highest expression possible because all things are possible when you focus on that.

Once I woke up to the tendencies of my ego, I knew I had no other option than to switch up the power differential. I knew it was the answer I had been seeking my entire life, but I could only see it when I was ready to see it. And it started with a bold lack of compassion and a solid drive to feel better in my life.

When I first started meditating, the ego was very much in dominance. The more I meditated and paid attention, the more I saw my little self and how much it was leading me away from being authentic. I thought it was the part of me that made me powerful, false. I thought it made me funny, false. I saw that it did not think twice about using intimidation to get what I wanted, true. I noticed its tendency to act from fear and then judge others for being fearful, true. I saw multiple tactics employed to ensure I did not feel the pain within myself or open my heart to those who I believed had wronged me, true and true.

Sitting still in silence with myself gave me a look at what was under the surface. Along with that, my commitment offered me experiences to feel the poison of jealousy, impatience, anger, and other emotions that I had kept myself from feeling in the past. I felt bad about feeling bad or mad and didn't know what to do with those emotions, so I did what many do, I stuffed them down. But through meditation and training my mind, I learned to remain still as they moved through me and used the perfect tool of breath to stay calm until the chaos passed. As I watched and felt like never before, it became clear that my actions, words, and thoughts did not always add to the world I dreamed of seeing. As clear as day, I was part of the problem, and my solution was to go deeper into my practice.

I sat despite how I was feeling. I felt despite the mental commentary. I relaxed despite the constriction, and as a result, I let go better and better each time. I got better at recognizing ego activation and practicing the pause to choose away from it. I began to see the ego in its small size, and it felt weaker than I remembered. I saw its strong preference that neither I nor anyone else meditates, ever. I saw its aversion to turning around and shining through the eye of wisdom. And I saw its distaste toward healing gatherings because it could not bear the risk of me experiencing a feeling of joining or a meditative state of oneness. The ego will take extraordinary measures to keep you out of the yoga studio and off the meditation cushion. And to overcome its guise, we must be awake to its resistance.

There are two states to navigate this life, sleeping or awake. To recognize the ego for what it is and take ownership of your power to train it is an essential rung on the awakening ladder. You will receive sudden ideas, great inspirations, and visions of your potential throughout your life. These are not by happenstance. These are meant for you. They come from you, and they warrant a discerning eye. Deep within each one of us, we know our dreams are possible. One of the most important things is to write them down. If you don't have a journal, get one. Writing down your dreams and desires gives proof of their existence. Do it before your ego finds out, dissuades you, and you forget your great inspiration, or worse, the universe passes it along to another who takes action and fulfills what you once dreamed.

After a decade of receiving and ignoring inspiration to practice meditation, I committed to sit. At first, I thought meditation would make me lose myself. I didn't believe I would be funny anymore. I feared it would make me weak and become one of those people who hug for too long. I worried that I wouldn't have the time, and I was petrified that I would not be good at it. But I knew I needed it in my life, so I cut some deals with the ego and devised a plan to use meditation to my advantage without letting go of anything that mattered to me.

I planned to decrease stress, manifest abundance, and not lose any of what made me cool. I was not interested in letting go of anything I enjoyed. I like controlling situations and people. I liked getting what I wanted and having better things than other people. I also enjoyed drinking three glasses of wine a night and popping the cork before noon on all holidays. I had no plans of letting go of my wine. I also remember telling MB that I didn't want to become fully enlightened because I wanted to come back to earth as a gorgeous singer like Faith Hill. The plan was good, one of my best yet. However, it was a plan that began to crumble from the very start. The absolute power of creating a relationship with my inner being was effortlessly crushing my ego agenda into sacred ash.

When Buddha was asked what he gained from meditation, he didn't recite a list of new qualities. Instead, he expressed everything he lost; anger, anxiety, depression, insecurity, fear of old age, and death. There was a period when every time I got into a car, I had an intense fear that I would be killed. There was a time in my life when I punched walls with a closed fist until my hand hurt so much I was able to cry. There were times in my life when I was consumed in the darkness of jealousy and unworthiness. And there were times in my life when I embodied the panic of financial ruin as my truth. To my unique degree, I lived what we have all lived, and when I woke up, I saw that it was all the orchestration of the ego. I have lived within separation and blindness that kept me from seeing the oneness of the energy that connects us. And perhaps the craziest aspect of living through the eyes of our small self is that it is our societal norm. It is supported, caressed, and encouraged. Also blamed, penalized, and rarely forgiven.

From the moment we come into this life, we are taught that we are separate through a series of labels and assignments. Boy or girl. Chubby or preemie. We are given a name and told who we take after. We are given a last name, certified, recorded, and put into a database. Figuratively and literally. We go into a system and are assigned a number to keep secret. It is instilled in us that the chances of someone stealing that number are high, and the consequences are significant. This is scary, and I know this concept contributed to a foundational mindset of fear for me. And the ego feasts on fear. Because it seems normal in our world to be on high alert, many feelings go unprocessed along our life journey. Unfortunately, we pass these characteristics and patterns onto our offspring and younger generations. And although the vast majority of parents, teachers, aunties, and uncles are well-intentioned, many of us learn at a very young age to push our emotions back down and endure pain without communication. Over time those feelings bubble up, and the ego's voice tells us that we are different for having ill feelings, but that's okay because we've got a pill for most of those feelings and the wiring that our brains have mapped. The ego further isolates us through the labels of our diagnosis and then cries sadness because we feel alone.

As long as we are in a body, we will experience the ego, but we can be free as we awaken to its games. I believe anyone who walks this path will find the same as Buddha. A loss of anger, anxiety, depression, insecurity, fear of old age, and death. I believe we can use our free will to remind the small self that although it is along for the ride, it will never get the keys. I believe we can create a relationship with the oneness that lives inside and allow our connected Self to have a more robust role in our lives.

We need roles to play and labels to function in this world. We need you to be the reader and me to be the author for this book to work. There is nothing wrong with the labels or our roles within them. We all play roles in this life, and I say, play those roles like you are going for an Academy Award, and then when you finish playing a role in your day, move on. As you aspire to this mindset, watch all beliefs around those roles being who you are, which means your attachment to those roles and your self-worth that may be tied up within them. Closely observe how you respond when your body is injured, and your sport is taken away. Closely watch when you achieve and do not achieve your goals. Closely monitor and fully feel how you process your life's experiences because your observances will tell you how much of your life is being lived by the ego, which believes that you are the roles you play.

The degree to which we suffer or succeed is within the understanding of our truth. We are spiritual beings living a human experience, and in our most exact nature, we are all-knowing, ever-powerful, and limitless. We are the big Self, the reflection of source energy in the buckets, and it is our birthright to make our minds one-pointed toward anything we desire in this life. Train the ego through the practice of meditation, live in an awake state, and you will discover a powerful teammate for life.

CHAPTER NINE

IT'S NOT ALL GOOD BUT IT ALL RESOLVES TO GOOD

"Your trials did not come to punish you but to awaken you."

Paramahansa Yogananada

I grew up in an "everything is going to be okay" household. It was not uncommon to have such an optimistic viewpoint as a part of my upbringing, and for the most part, it appeared to hold. I had not experienced a significant tragedy or trauma for four-plus decades, save a few broken bones and grandparent funerals. I give thanks for this profusely, and my family unit talks about this often when we are together. "We are so blessed," we say. All five of us are alive and marginally scathed by life.

But, in light of events I experienced in recent years, I question, had everything been okay? Or did this belief gloss over decades of emotional suppression that seriously compromised my point of attraction?

Was not the fear I experienced whenever I got into a car a byproduct of unresolved trauma? Have I not existed my entire life suppressing mental impressions of violence from the news and irrevocable imprints of animal and human cruelty? Have reports of motorists plowing down groups of cyclists and gunmen with murderous intent taking the lives of others kept me on high alert for exceptional danger?

And what about all the things I have done willingly, like watching psychologically thrilling movies or horror flicks that have encouraged gray matter growth in my amygdala? Has not all this manifested into deeply patterned defense mechanisms and psychic numbness that help get me out of bed each day and walk the streets at night?

And where does a soul's journey fit in here? If it is true that we are eternal beings, then what in the heck kind of history did we bring into this world? And have we forgiven and been forgiven? Do I have outstanding debts to pay? Do you?

We pay money to watch terror play out on the big screen. We dress in team colors and paint our faces to show allegiance while our players assert repeated trauma on each other's bodies. We consistently build tension in our systems by putting ourselves in front of violent behavior and communication that we call the news. And by societal standards, it is normal, but it is also what we habitually deny; repeated trauma to our system.

Let's take another example, something I learned in my advanced studies massage program while taking a Trauma

And The Body course. Our intellect knows that on Tuesday at 11:00 am, we are going into an outpatient clinic for a minor and routine procedure that will require only a local anesthetic. To the intellect, which understands there's much worse out there in the world, this is not a big deal, especially since it is so common for people's health status to require regular and routine procedures. But to the nervous system, it is a life or death situation, and with the first incision, the threat becomes realized. If we are not honoring this truth by engaging in regular practices that balance our nervous system, the fight or flight center will continue to expand as we soldier on through life suppressing the traumas of our reality.

Alone and left to fester, these compounded traumas rest in our tissues while a portion of our vibration tunes to darkness. As this resonance is not immune to the law of attraction, we steer ourselves toward our greatest fears. Circumstances in life will arise that match our shadows within. Although these experiences give us the opportunity to overcome trauma and heal our samskaras, most people will cower and cling to what they know in the face of fear. Because our world does not educate us on the importance of knowing and tuning the energy body, we end up making what we do not want a part of our future identity.

I commonly hear identity-minded phrases like "my anxiety," "my fear," "my depression," "my inability to relax," and "my busy mind." In the process of fueling these words with our attention, we negate the truth of our most natural vibration and deny what Dr. Wayne Dyer said time and again, that we don't attract what we want; we attract what we are. We live behind labels that help us understand our position in the world despite how small they make us feel, and we drive ourselves out of alignment from our center and into the grips of the ego.

As I observe the world and the unrest that persists, I see a great deal of fear at the source of our worldly existence. And if there is any energy MB warns me to stay out of its fear. He explains that fear will attract the exact thing that we are fearing or its equal. By practicing the pause and backing away from consensus fear, we begin to regain control and heal the darkness that attracts us to fearful experiences. We heal when we live awake to the ego rule of separation and feel all experiences within conscious mind activation. And when we heal, the world heals because our energy in each moment affects the whole.

There is heaven on this earth and hell on this earth. There is the lightest of light and the darkest of dark. The truth of this world means that people will be murdered today, and some will lose their minds to jealousy and derangement today. Some children will become gravely ill today, and millions of animals will receive abuse today. Babies will be born into extreme poverty, oppression, and violence today. And people who carry burdens of unresolved pain will end their life each and every day. These are our sisters and brothers, manifestations of the same cosmic force. Our essence is exact, and whether we like it or not, we are a global family. Contrary to what I used to believe, there is no *my* or *your* suffering. There is only our suffering. We are deeply connected, and through life's challenges and traumas, we receive opportunities to transform that suffering.

Regardless of how society labels traumas and conditions in life, the awake athlete remembers the expanded view which serves the collective. Instead of finding victim and victimizer in the storylines, we see karmic alignment and opportunities to heal. This way, no one is condemned. Our brothers and sisters are free to evolve and experience redemption. We do not have to agree with the gunman or the drunk driver's behavior because their actions are not okay. But, if we are to advance in our spiritual growth, we must unlock our constricted hearts, feel the pain we are carrying, and become vulnerable in the face of this fear-based world to see that our safety lies in our defenselessness.

As our commit to sit practice grows stronger, we learn to let life move through us and us through it with more ease. Then, as we navigate terrible races, heartbreaking relationships, fear-inducing tragedies, and the deathly aftermaths of natural disasters, we naturally release our attachment to the ego's need for things to be different and are free to focus on the processing of life's events. We have the power to focus on the expansive vision and the soul's journey while honoring the human experience.

According to Patanjali, the way life bumps us around on this planet is so that we finally say "no more." It's the moment we decide to change the way we play the game of life once and for all. BJ and I call it the "sucks enough" moment. I hit it somewhere in my late twenties, and that is when I started to open to another way of living. And although pain brings us to this moment, it is quite refreshing because once we say "no more" and mean it, we awaken. Awakening is an ongoing birth that can feel breech at times. Although smooth in its intelligence, it can rip you to shreds. But it's the recognition that life may tear us to shreds and the vulnerability of showing up in shreds that paints the masterpiece of our lives and allows us to learn how to play this game of life with utter acceptance. Acceptance is the absence of resistance, it is neutral, and neutrality is not apathy. It is caring profoundly and feeling deeply, without attachment. It is a perspective that is woke to this earth school and accepts that every day is a new lesson in the current chapter of life. Acceptance is a necessary step in welcoming all things.

If I'm to be fully honest, for most of my life, my reality felt more like a streak of fortune that had yet to run out. And isn't that fear itself? I did not understand the soul's journey as I do today. I did not know that earth is a school, and we are presented with daily teachings relevant to our growth. I did not understand that when Sir Isaac Newton discovered every action has an equal and opposite reaction, that also pertained to me and how I move through the world. I did not have knowledge of universal law, vibrational alignment, or the suffering allowed under the watchful eye of unconditional love. And I certainly didn't comprehend unconditional love as I do now, nor have I ever been called to such incredible heights of it as I did in the year 2021.

But before I go down that road, I'd be remiss not to point out

that just because you choose to live an awake life does not mean
the waves of life are stopping. And no Friday or vacation in this
life will make them stop. You may feel like you are drowning
at times while other times you surf the heck out of whatever
comes your way, but regardless of the feels, you will be further
on your spiritual journey and wiser for it in the end. To what
degree depends on how willing you are to stay awake when
everything screams, "go back to sleep!"

This book is the one I felt my entire life, and I promise you
the resistance to get it to where it is today feels like a lifetime's
worth. But if you are reading this, I'm on the other side of that
now. And I attribute much of my perseverance and strength to
a soul-purifying trauma I experienced. My story has changed.
It now includes proximity to violence that I never imagined
for my life and serious healing that I would otherwise not have
chosen on my own.

The following recount is mine. It is my experience, and it is true
for me only.

I dedicate this book to Mary, who, on February 13, 2021, was
murdered by her ex-boyfriend, who then killed himself. It
happened in the home they previously shared less than one
mile from my home as I sat in the deep peace of meditation
while the sun set serenely on the day. When I became aware of
her passing and the earliest details of the crime the following
morning, it was evident that my meditation timed perfectly with
the moments before and throughout her death. This alignment
stunned my human self, honored the innate intelligence that

pulled me to the cushion that day and connected me to her transition that only the divine would orchestrate.

Although there was no palpable connection to Mary during that meditation, I experienced a rush of peace, a state I had not felt in the previous few months. My meditations were messy leading up to that day. My sleep was disruptive, nightmares were terrifyingly realistic, and I suffered an odd bout of frequent headaches, all of which ceased that Saturday evening around sunset. I was aware of a disturbance in the field leading up to this day and a feeling of dread that I could not shake until those moments when I resided in peace and Mary transitioned into the same.

My spiritual self reminds me often that the result of this entanglement, or murder-suicide as the police and press refer to it, was a karmic collision of two souls that no one could have prevented. Mary and I often talked about the karmic contract of her relationship with him. We talked about how the sun shined on them both the same, but that truth didn't mean she had to stay in the relationship. Mary knew she was not responsible for his happiness, and we talked about her home environment being stronger than her will. She was awake to the precariousness of her situation, and I don't believe that she was living in fear, but, as I know now, she was only sharing a degree of her true reality with me.

I worked closely with Mary when she left this earth and had been for the previous three years. We shared in morning rituals just the day before, sipping delicious coffee from a local roastery and selecting tribal medicine cards as our guide for the day. When I look back on the cards she chose that morning, I see her fate was hovering close by. She had gone down a road too far for too long. There was no other way out for her soul, and I have a deep sense that her tragic exit was the last piece she needed to be free of the pain she endured.

Mary was a natural-born awake athlete; she was drawn to mastery and serving others. She exemplified these qualities through endurance sports, as an athlete and a coach, as a veterinarian, and in her death, a place most will overlook. Throughout our years together, she called me to a level of merit I would not have sought without her. It seems now Mary was the teacher playing the role of my student. It was 2017 when she chose me as her guide on the spiritual path; from that moment forward, I knew to put that role above all else with her, and I am so glad I did.

I believe Mary came to this earth to get the spark; I witnessed her find it and light it aflame. I watched her move mountains on her journey to live in the vulnerability and truth she so deeply desired, two components of her life that we talked about in our very first and very last meeting. Our sessions had the potential to run deep. Mary was open to healing, and like everything she endeavored, she was willing to do what it took to heal her soul.

Mary battled the same battle of dark and light that we all struggle with in life. She fought unworthiness and knew that love was the answer. There were moments in the last year of her life when I held her hand and reminded her that she was loved and that she was love, and in her deepest core, she knew this to be true. We discussed the truth of what was presented in their relationship as love and she was clear that their path together was not a joyous one. I helped her hatch more than one plan to leave him, and each time those plans fell apart, I asked her why she chose to stay. "I don't know," she would tell me, but now I do. The darkness was proving powerful, and the environment of her home was dim. It had all become more potent than her will. I've heard that the web of a black widow spider is chaotic and extremely sticky. It's hard to free yourself once you are caught up in it. This is the only way I can describe what I now believe Mary returned to every time she walked into their home.

I often sought counsel with non-physical support and MB, which allowed me to stay on task and be there for her uniquely to our soul contract. There were countless times when I wanted to save her, shake her, and scream, but more so, I wanted so badly to just be her friend. Being her guide felt too much to bear. Sometimes, I just wanted to open a bottle of wine and watch Netflix with her for days. There was a part of me that wanted the relationship I saw others having with her, but Mary and I knew that was not our partnership on this earth, not in this life.

I had known Mary for 15 years at the time of her death. We met through Nicole DeBoom's Skirts Sports Entourage ambassador program when BJ and I lived in Boulder. Nicole had just won IRONMAN Wisconsin in the first skirt prototype, and her Entourage was about to come into form. Mary and I would both be selected as the first generation of Skirts. We first met via Facebook and then in person at IRONMAN Coeur d'Alene 2008. We stayed in each other's awareness throughout the years and connected again in the physical at IRONMAN Lake Placid 2015. At this point, Mary was on a quest to qualify for the IRONMAN World Championship held each year in Kailua, Kona. She placed 9th in her age group in Lake Placid, but a championship qualification required higher placement that day. However, Mary did qualify later that year with an age group podium at IRONMAN Arizona, which led us to connect again after she raced the 2016 world championship. BJ and I were living on the road, and it worked perfectly to meet up in Arizona, where she lived at the time to record an episode of the YogiTriathlete podcast. We titled it "Mary Knott On Finding Kona." Slowly, our lives were merging into physical alignment again, and then, in 2017, she wrote an email to BJ and me titled "Thoughts."

I hope you don't think I'm crazy for reaching out but I think things happen for a reason, and over the last few months I've been feeling really strongly that I need more of what you have to offer in my life. Specifically—plant-based diet and meditation/mindfulness.

Would you ever consider letting me come visit for a few days and just be immersed in your lifestyle? I would pay you-- I would love to do yoga, do some mindfulness/meditation work, cook together and talk about plant-based nutrition and maybe BJ would let me tag along on some training too during that time? I can get a hotel or whatever nearby. I know I'm basically inviting myself... :) I don't want to do it

remotely- I know you offer that, but I feel like I would need to really
step away from my life and the stress/obligations at home to really
absorb what you can teach me. Let me know your thoughts.

Mary

I responded to Mary and explained that her timing could not
be more, well, timely. BJ and I had been talking about a
48-hour retreat where people could fully immerse themselves
into a high vibrational life with us in Carlsbad. Mary came on
her first High Vibe Retreat in the fall of 2017 and returned for
another three, always bringing friends to share in the light that
danced brightly around her.

Shortly after her first retreat, Mary asked me to guide her
on the road to enlightenment. I use the word enlightenment
specifically because I am clear that was her goal. Mary was all
in from the start. Anyone who knew her is not surprised to read
this. She knew how to train the body, she had a strong desire to
train the mind, and when Mary saw something she wanted, she
would not stop until she got it. And I do not doubt that she is
further along the path now for the life she lived on earth.

Mary was one of the most generous people I have ever known.
When Clark ate a dish towel and ended up in the emergency
vet to the tune of almost $8,000, I woke up the following day to
$1,000 from Mary in our PayPal account. There are a hundred
more Mary stories just like this one because she was not just
generous with material things; she was generous with her heart
and soul. I had the pleasure of guiding some of her athletes in

mindset training, and they always shared how supportive she was anytime one of them came to her with a hair-brained idea for an epic adventure. She was the supporter of all supporters. Mary's ability to care for others far surpassed many people on this earth, and in the end, her kind heart kept someone in her life who fell so far into darkness that he took her life along with his own.

I desire this chapter not to pin Mary in the victim role and perpetuate a residing belief that bad things happen to good people. Instead, I invite you to dive under the surface of what appears to be real because I believe Mary is calling us to awaken our minds, open our hearts and consider not just the headline but the journey of a soul without judgment. Judgment was a significant theme in my work with Mary; like many of us, she did not want to be judged. She was frightened of being judged, so we could honor her now by not condemning her to the powerlessness of victimhood.

Four days before her death, BJ and I had our bi-monthly session with MB, which also was the same day as the final session I shared with Mary in my home. At one point, MB looked directly at me and told me that there is no death and I needed to focus on eternal life. It sent a chill up my spine. The week prior, I had a dream about a person holding BJ and a woman in an apartment, and he was going to kill them. I was looking in from the outside, and I could not get inside to save them. Then, two nights before her murder, BJ dreamed of a woman drowning in a river, and when he tried to save her, she said, "I'm already gone."

I share these remembrances not as a compelling way to evoke drama but to present a clear picture of the knowledge of our higher selves. When I woke up to the news early Sunday morning that she had been killed by the man she said she did not fear, I was bombarded with the meaning of everything I felt leading up to that day, and it pounded me into all of my survival mechanisms as a human. I knew that I would heal because I live with the grace of the universe as my lead, but I also knew this would be the greatest challenge of my life.

Grace can be defined as the refinement of movement. Likewise, the path of awakening is the fine-tuning of consciousness. As I intertwine these concepts, I have realized a masterful yet ongoing recovery from an experience that shook me like nothing else. It blew open my vault of suppression, and when this opening occurred, the energy that bound me so close to this darkness was free to move. I felt so much, and it came in intense waves, but I knew too much not to allow for it all. So I allowed, and I felt, and it was all the feels.

Anger. Anger at Mary, anger at him, anger at me. Anger that she kept so much from me and so angry that I could not meditate as I did before. MB said that bringing this level of darkness into my meditation would not be good, and therefore he instructed me to stop meditating. At first, this was a relief because closing my eyes was intensely scary, but after a few weeks, I just felt angry about it.

Humility. Humility that my life continues and that I was chosen to lead her on the spiritual path. And humility for all I am learning as she further thins the veil of delusion for me.

Fear. This was so immense. Fear in the final few weeks when they were still alive, and he was becoming unhinged. Fear because he knew where we lived and fear because he had been in my home. Fear that he knew I was guiding her to a life without him and fear that I was not safe. Fear that I would never be safe. Fear that electrocuted my body for days after hearing the news. It was months before I returned to wearing an eye mask for sleeping which I've done for as long as I can remember. The twinkle of light on the ceiling that creeps through our bedroom curtains at night was no longer an annoyance but a welcomed friend. I questioned the black-out nature of those curtains more than once. I clung to daylight and dreaded the setting sun. I went everywhere with my husband by my side and wondered if I would ever be able to be alone in the dark again. Yet throughout the paralyzing fear, I also felt deep compassion arising, and I knew I was being taught something that I would use to assist others in the future.

Neediness. Are people mad at me? Am I being judged? Why isn't anyone asking how I am doing? Don't they know I live a mile from the crime scene? Why don't they care about me? Why are they not including me? Don't they know I was in danger too?

Am I being judged? Oh my God, what if I am judged?

The ego flailed in a sea of emotion. I watched closely as the waves built and crashed, sometimes taking my breath away entirely and other times ending in deep sobs of letting go. I leaned into my husband, and he into me. I felt our relationship strengthen. I talked with awake souls close to me and felt their selfless embrace meet me exactly where I was, inviting me to do the same for myself. To those enlightened teachers and dear friends near and far who urged me to stay awake, I am forever changed by your divine guidance.

I observed that the initial phase of trauma and tragedy is an ego-less state. It is a time of no words and no judgment. A time of shock, awe, and unconditional support between a collective of individuals now bonded for life. It is an inconceivable pause in the ever-moving time-space reality of our lives. But with time, the reemergence of the ego became evident.

The neediness, fear, and anger were all there to remind me that the "I" part of me was injured and desperately seeking a return to a time that felt like it did before he did that to her. Of course, this is not possible, but the ego will convince you that you will never be as happy or whole as you were before the trauma. This is a lie.

As the ego reared its narrow-minded vision, I watched people debate about moving forward vs. moving on. I worried about doing it the right way. I watched judgments fly around how people expressed their process, and some of those came from within me. I felt dismissed and yet understood. I watched the ego celebrate its position in the drama. I lived in a washing machine of contrasting emotions and prayed daily for the strength to honor it all. I watched the mind closely and saw its constant demand for more information. Particularly in those initial days and weeks, I watched my mind receive information and desire more, even when it invited more fear and darkness. I watched it search for a solution to a life situation that can never be resolved on the human level.

I lived what I knew, that left to its own devices, the mind will never be satisfied. The more it knew, the more it wanted. I witnessed my mind wanting more details about the crime and the crime scene, from investigative findings to things that no one but Mary knew. I watched my imagination conjure horrifying visions of the evil in his eyes and the terror in hers. I felt deeply saddened over their animals and what they may have seen. It was a relentless brigade of thoughts that made me shutter and mental images that kept me up at night.

But staying awake allowed me to watch how my mind continually sought, received, and demanded more, no matter how much it compounded the trauma. It stirred up questions I never thought I would ask, but on top of this tremendous loss, I could not deny that Mary was helping me reach a new level of controlling my mind. I was, as MB said, called off the bench like when Krishna commands Arjuna in the Gita to stand up and fight amid utter despair. He told me to watch very closely where my mind was going and to use my strength to focus on life, not death.

There were so many times that I did not want to be where I was standing. I wanted to go to sleep and relive the horror that took Mary away because misery and fear felt like the easier choice. But I knew I did not have the luxury of that choice. Not me, anyhow. Not on my chosen path and the knowledge I have gained from what I traversed in life. And indeed, I did not have that choice because Mary was my student, and she was asking me to live what I teach. I felt incredibly alone as a human and fully supported in my spiritual development. I chose to lean into the latter and witness the former. I feel like I earned a Ph.D. in my truth as a spirit living a human experience, and there is no doubt it was my next step on the path. This trauma was the catalyst for my existence's most significant spiritual growth spurt, an awakening like none I had experienced before. From the moment I heard the fateful news, I felt Mary's call to see this through the eyes of truth, the quality we spoke of countless times, meditated upon hundreds of times, and visualized for her life in our final times together.

I've heard that everything we experience prepares us for the next thing, and I know that the prior decade of my life prepared me for this. Getting to know the witness part of me through daily meditation practice and experiencing that powerful pause every day has provided me with a spacious seat to receive the divine sequence of life.

Just three months before Mary, my mother-in-law, Teri, suddenly and unexpectedly transitioned from the earth. Teri exemplified selfless service and unconditional love. BJ and I recognized quickly that these were the teachings she left for us to carry on, and we dedicated ourselves to her legacy. During this time, we went deep with Meditator Bob to learn more about the death of our bodies, the release of our souls, and the unrestricted flow of unconditional love. And so, at the beginning of 2021, a few months after Teri left her body, I declared two things about my life and how I intended to live in the coming year. First, to increase the vibrancy of my life so I made some dietary shifts, like reducing excess salt, oil, and processed foods. I also took to a deeper study and practice of Ayurveda[17] to optimize my health.

The second intention for 2021 was unconditional love, a declaration that is helping me to emerge from Mary's death as a more compassionate and loving being. It is so clear that my mother-in-law brought this to light with how she lived, and Mary accelerated this calling through her death, but no one has asked more of me in this way than Mary's murderer.

As spring emerged, the days from February 13th became calculations by month. Time moved forward without apology, and still, the drop pin of that Saturday evening, although further away, still feels like a moment ago. I can go there. I can go there so quickly and not miss a detail.

I hear the horrifying words and guttural tone of our friend's voice repeatedly cry out, "He killed her! He killed her! And then he killed himself!" And it brings me right back. Right into the depths of the moment when I realized a permanence that made my blood turn cold. A recognition of unthinkable violence and the instant sickness that overcame my being.

---

17 Ayurveda is the sister science to yoga. It is ancient Indian medicine with roots as deep as the supreme science of yoga. The base of Ayurvedic understanding is that when balance is present, health and healing ensue. Ayurvedic treatment includes medicinal herbs, lifestyle behavior, massage, and yoga to support the body's natural healing mechanisms.

It is an undeniable weight of truth that life as you know it
has changed forever because someone you love in this life
will never be in physical form again. At first, my mind just
replayed traumatic visions of when I heard the news and
what happened in the apartment that night. I was repeatedly
traumatized multiple times a day. It was a system overload
like I had never experienced before, and within it, I knew the
only choice was to remain awake and feel it all. So I turned
to the highest vibrational foods. I turned to my sister, who is a
trauma therapist, and my family. I walked with BJ and Clark
close by my side, and I began documenting my 15-year journey
with Mary in my journal. And for months, my processing and
healing did not include him. It couldn't; I wasn't ready.

In early April of 2021, I was preparing to leave for a yoga
retreat I was hosting in Costa Rica when I received a *knowing* to
start down the path of forgiveness. I felt a purity in my heart,
and it tasked me to surround his soul in light and pray for his
way forward in a world where so few will do the same. And
although it would be so easy in the short term to dismiss this
man, I know that is not the path forward because it is not, as
the yogis say, *right action* to do so. As I heal my soul contract
with Mary, I also heal the one I had with a man once named
Hilton "Willie" Williams. It's bigger than the pain he carried in
this life and the evil that reigned dominant that evening. It's his
path forward as a soul and mine, for that sake. He faces a long
and arduous road ahead because he violated the principle of
ahimsa to the most extreme degree. But source light still shines
on his soul the same, and so I know that light is the only path
forward for me.

IT'S NOT ALL GOOD BUT IT ALL RESOLVES TO GOOD

To close my heart and reduce this soul to human behavior is to deny my essence and divine right to be good. All beings must pay their karmic debts. It is not my position to pass judgment or enforce retribution. It is my job to forgive so that I may heal, so that they may heal, so that we may all heal because, as interconnected beings, there is only collective suffering. So when my mind takes me down the trauma replay road, which pins her as the powerless victim and he as the evil victimizer, I turn my attention to the ancient Ho'Oponopono prayer. A prayer to "make things right." It consists of four simple statements, and when recited and felt with intention, gives power to right all wrongs, resolve the unresolvable and replace darkness with light.

I love you.

I'm sorry.

Please forgive me.

Thank you.

As you say these statements, either silently or aloud, it is essential to feel them and allow any emotion to arise without denial. Hold the person or circumstance in your mind's eye and recite this prayer five times in tribute to them, followed by an additional three times in homage to yourself. Do this until you feel calm and return to this prayer often and always when you catch yourself seeing the world's circumstances through the separate eyes of the ego.

And so, amidst hefty impulses to get caught up in the horror flick that became reality, especially in those first few weeks, I followed a simple recipe; feel it all, deny nothing, and let it go. Over and over again.

To feel sad and be awake.

To feel depressed and be awake.

To feel angry and be awake.

To feel non-forgiving and be awake.

To feel scared and be awake.

To feel judged and be awake.

To feel absolutely furious and be awake.

To forgive and be awake.

Even though this world can be one of misery, and it will bring us to our knees more than once, I know we can live with reverence amid the darkness. I know we can laugh in joyful expression and trust that everything is in order. I know we can see the loving truth beyond disturbance and choose it in the face of egoic condemnation. Making this choice is not an easy option because staying awake is not the popular choice, and we may be judged for it, but like the sages and yogis have told us for thousands of years, the road to awakening is not for the faint of heart.

For my life experience, there is no time before this trauma ever again, and there is no earth that includes Mary in the role that she played for 44 years and two months, but I am still here, and I have a purpose of continuing my awakening. So therefore, I have one choice: to live the teachings I shared with her over the years because they are the keys to the kingdom where her blessed soul now resides.

Three months after Mary left this earth, I received the following message.

Hey you,
I want you to know that your friend did not die in vain.

I truly believe that if I wasn't in your group, I would still be in a very toxic relationship where I would say 80% of my friends continued to be concerned that he was going to kill me.

I believe your friend actually saved my life.

For this message, the enormous healing I have embraced, and the capacity of love I now know, I stand in faith that although not all is good in this world, it always resolves to good.

CHAPTER TEN

ENLIGHTENED PERFORMANCE

*"Be watchful—the grace of God appears suddenly,
it comes without warning to an open heart."*

Rumi

I wore bib number 1039 as I screamed down route 73 into
Keene, NY, on my Kestrel 4000 triathlon bike. The Adirondack
skies put on a grand show that day. Lightning bolts cut through
black clouds illuminating the ominous backdrop. Thunder
rumbled the earth, and my body shook so severely from the
cold that my shoes unclipped from the pedals. My brake pads
were rendered mute by the relentless downpour of rain that
blanketed the area. I heard later that race officials pulled 700
participants from Mirror Lake that morning. Swimming was
never much of an issue for me, so I had well cleared the timing
mat when the weather moved in. Instead, at that time, I was
descending the most technical section of the IRONMAN Lake
Placid bike course amid a mountain storm.

"I am heat; I give and withhold the rain. I am immortality and I am death; I am what is and what is not".

These verses from the Gita pulsed through my mind. Anything can happen, I thought. I could die. I could survive. I could quit. I could keep going. I could relax, and I could trust. I could trust in the energy that was behind it all.

I focused my vision as best I could and held on as I let go. As I relaxed within the intensity of my circumstance, a peace came over me. I realized that I was okay with living or dying. I was okay with making it down the hill or crashing. I was okay that the conditions were beyond my control, and I was at peace because I was in surrender, a concept I previously considered to be a sign of weakness. But in those moments, it felt more like a level of bravery far above what I had reached before.

I was in God's hands, and I felt safer there than in my own. I kept returning to the experience of the present moment and seeing that I was safe. Every moment I checked in, I was safe. Albeit cold and drenched but none of those things meant dead. Every time I checked in, I was alive, and in circumstances like that storm, being alive meant I had no problems.

After what felt like hours, but perhaps was just twenty or so minutes, I reached the bottom of the descent and approached an aid station. My eyes focused on a port-a-john, which looked like an oasis that day, a shelter to get warm. I slowed my bike, and a volunteer ran to my side. Apparently, I looked as terrible as I felt. He helped me disembark my 48-inch stallion that

somehow remained upright on the downhill and delivered me
to that moment safely.

The volunteer redirected me to the aid station tent, where I
was given a chair to rest, a trash bag to wear, and latex gloves to
warm my hands. My body shook violently from the cold, more
so than when I was riding. The safety of my reality allowed my
body to release fully, so I stayed in a state of surrender and let it
shake. From time to time, I steadied myself to not fall out of my
chair; otherwise, I let my body do what it needed to do.

As time passed, more and more athletes joined me under
the tent. From super-fit experienced triathletes to first-timers
getting baptized into long-course triathlon, our differences did
not matter. No one cared about political affiliations or if we
had ever cut someone off in traffic. What we cared about was
each other. So we gathered closely, body to body, human to
human, all grateful for being safe. We lent words of support
to one another and expressed gratitude to the volunteers who
offered us layers of their clothing for our recovery.

In moments like these, with eyes wide open, we see and feel the
unity of life. It is a state that we can always reside within and
the very one that connects us to all that is, was, and ever will
be. It is an optimal state of being for training and racing and
one that will become second nature as you choose to stay the
course. It will not remove life's challenges, but it will connect
you to a deep awareness of Self where witnessing our outer and
inner world becomes the default that forever places us within a
position of power.

As time continued to tick away under the tent that day, the inevitable questions began to surface. How could I go on? I had 90 miles left to ride and a marathon to run. How would it be possible to recover and tackle all that lay ahead? There was no evidence that I would be able to leave that aid station in anything but a car. I thought of BJ, who was spectating on account of an injury that kept him from lining up with me that day. I thought of my in-laws, who traveled up from Massachusetts to see us both race. Quitting seemed out of reach but getting back on my bike to finish the race felt further. I wondered if they were worried. I didn't want them to worry.

My mind spiraled from the safety of presence to the darkness of despair. It was doubting one moment and determined the next. My awareness ping-ponged from my lower to higher self, but I was in the gap, watching and knowing that what I was learning was patience and what I was feeling was the grace of the universe at my side. The very same grace that has since become the lead in my life, and at that moment, I knew anything was possible. I had 17 hours to finish the race. All I needed to do was be in the moment I was in, nowhere else. My meditation practice was right there for me, offering calm in the chaos. Unlike the fleeting nature of motivation, my awake athlete self showed up as an unshakeable resource.

I waited with a depth of patience that was new to me as I continued to watch the mind, sip electrolytes, and take in nutrition to fuel the momentum of my desire to finish the race. I visualized the finish line I had spent the previous nine months preparing for and gave my body the time it needed to find homeostasis again. Then, about 30 minutes later, a switch flipped. I stood up and announced, "I'm good, oh my God, I'm good. I'm outta here".

I wished the others well and rode away with my gorgeous Sunrise triathlon kit from Smashfest Queen covered in a heavy-duty trash bag and my hands comforted in latex. I was optimistic, but never more so than when not even five minutes after leaving the aid station did another competitor pass me and say, "look, over there." I followed his gesture to see a patch of cerulean sky break through the gray; I pedaled the remaining distance with a renewed sense of joy. That day I realized a personal best IRONMAN time, my fastest marathon to date, and the most "best kit" comments ever. Indeed it was a great kit.

There gets to be a time on the awake athlete path when you really begin to experience life as it is, and this was one of those experiences. I had so many reasons to fight the conditions on the day. I could have lingered in fear of what may come next. But instead, I chose faith, and it was not blind. It was faith in the very thing I had been communing with in meditation for almost four years. And I believed, with my entire being, that my experience would not be cut short by quitting. This was not positive thinking; it was a product of the work I had done on my meditation cushion day after day, and that day, it showed up effortlessly for me.

With time, we get better in the practice. We learn to let go of how circumstances have to play out and turn our focus to our response to how life is playing out. It's not a denial of the dissatisfied voice or negative thoughts which come from the ego. It's a practice of feeling and letting go. I mean, it was certainly not pleasant to be that cold and that wet, but by witnessing instead of indulging that voice, I remained in control. I starved fear-based impulses and unsatisfied mental preferences, and by doing so, I guided myself towards an enlightened state of being, where I accepted what was and what could be without a fight.

As I recall, this was the first time I truly surrendered my will to the greater will of the divine. Circumstances were out of my hands, and to a large degree, that made surrender easy. However, I've come to know that we can practice this beautiful art without circumstances becoming dire. Surrender is a profound experience that occurs when we lighten up our grip on life and realize that it is not all up to us. We do not have to make anything happen. We do not have to force. We do not have to live with anxiety, impatience, worry, or fear. These are calling cards of the ego that says we are all alone on our path in life. And although only you can walk your path, and only I can walk mine, we are never alone because it is impossible to be alone. We are intelligently connected with all life, and non-physical support surrounds us in a field of limitless possibility. At our core, we are the energy of pure potentiality, the same as the pure consciousness from which we came. And in surrender, we lean into this stream of potential where all things are possible, and it is here that we enter powerful states for performance.

If we resist events in our life because we believe things should be another way, we deny our power to choose flow. When we act from the energy of resistance, we create from the energy of resistance. This magnetizes us to draw more circumstances into our reality that will call us to resist. I observe this regularly in the lives of athletes, and I see it because I have navigated it in my own life experience.

Only when we stop fighting the cicumstances of the now moment will flow become a part of our norm. Until then, we can feel trapped in resistant response cycles that move us further from enlightened performance. If we can keep leaning into life with a calmer mind, we'll grow out of the need to fight so much and into way of being where we are free to enter flow. Over all we'll be much better at feeling life's rolls and punches, delights, and detours without so much struggle. And we will gain clarity that the ego's need to control is the exact reason why something extraordinary has not arisen.

As we sit our fit butts down onto the meditation cushion and turn our attention inwards, we learn that a cavern of non-resistant energy flows deep to all that is. And when we can find rest amid intensity, we know our performance is becoming enlightened.

Athletes have a common saying, get comfortable with the uncomfortable, and I agree with this, but most athletes engage in this practice from a state of fight and dissatisfaction. Instead of relaxation and acceptance. We grit through the workout to show ourselves that we can keep moving when it is painful.

We endure the mind's impulses screaming for us to stop and tell ourselves that we are stronger than the pain. This works, absolutely it works, but it is a heavy way. Let me give you an example of this from my training history. Those of you familiar with the training ground of Boulder, Colorado, are then familiar with the iconic Old Stage climb. My first triathlon coach used to have me do Old Stage repeats, and the mantra I used to conquer those repeats was, "I'm a bigger bitch than this hill." Although successful and accurate at the time, the mantra was exhaustive and resistant.

I've since found another way. It's lighter and less effortful; it says that all we encounter along our way holds life lessons, not misfortunes. There is wisdom to gain from all experiences. It is a way of being that contains an inner knowing that we are never victims of our circumstances and that although there will be many intense climbs in our life, there is a way to go about them that lessens our suffering, which in turn reduces the collective suffering. It's the one that requires the ego to be the servant and not the master. It's the one that always asks our hearts to be open and relaxed. It's the one that recognizes that there are bigger hands at play at all times, and surrendering into those hands is to become the power of them. It is the natural evolution of one who practices the science of the mind by walking the path of yoga.

It is quite interesting how it all comes together in this existence—interconnected limitless souls on eternal journeys that have landed here on earth to live a human experience through a physical body hardwired for survival. We all have an instinctual spark to fight and we will never lose our innate drive to survive. However, as neuroscience has proven, the gray matter in our amygdala is far beyond what is necessary for mere survival and that is compromising our ability to realize our potential. There will be pain on this path, that is for sure, but consider this, it is not the pain that causes us to suffer—it is our fight against the pain that is the creator of misery.

The path to enlightened performance creates space between the impulses of resistance and our response to the resistance. As we become aware and back away from the unnecessary fight, we tune ourselves to navigating life as it is without judgment. With less energy going to the battle of that which we cannot change, we harness more power towards what we can change. This is yoking and steering our minds like masters.

Mastery is a present state where intuitive knowledge of what to do and when to do it can be heard. It's a moment-to-moment process in which wisdom flows into action, and the more moments of mastery we sew together, the more time we spend in optimal states of consciousness. And it is my surmise that optimal states of consciousness are not different from optimal states of athletic performance. Mastery is not exclusive to a class or race of people. It is not reserved for those with ivy league diplomas or worldly success. Many very smart people in this world are far from reaching levels of mastery. Mastery is formless and never out of stock. There is nothing to hoard. It is there for you and me, non-discriminate. It is timeless and ageless, all-knowing and unlimited. It is pure alignment with your awake athlete within.

Enlightened performance is a state of mastery. It is a state of unshakeable calm that permeates all life circumstances, especially amid chaos in the body, mind, or external surroundings. It is a frequency of attunement that entrusts unconditional love and limitless potential of the unseen as the predominant guide in athleticism. It is a recognition that the energy that creates worlds is the essence of who you are, and when in alignment with that energy, nothing is off the table.

CHAPTER ELEVEN

THE TIME IS NOW

"Time isn't precious at all, because it is an illusion. What you perceive as precious is not time but the one point that is out of time: the Now. That is precious indeed. The more you are focused on time—past and future—the more you miss the Now, the most precious thing there is."

Ekhart Tolle

As I move into the final week of 2021, I find myself titrating a load of ego-induced anxiety to meet my goal of finishing this book draft before midnight on the 31st with the knowledge that I undoubtedly will. I am being relentlessly gentle as I yoke the ego and steadily move towards my goal. I get better and better every day as it attempts to pressurize the expression of this creation. I am going easy with myself, and as the seabirds teach, I am resting in the storm's eye as it rages around me. The more I relax into it and allow for it, the easier it is to let go and move forward.

This is me living awake, and I am always in practice. I share my experiences with you because I am not beyond the techniques or studies I write about in this book. I am living them daily and finding them increasingly more potent while my effort feels far less. My life is a moment-to-moment practice of everything within the covers of this book. I anchor in the present moment, where I get to be deliberate in how I live my life. I have stayed devoted to my practice since the start and understand that the comfort of my life is here for me to go deeper. And that requires me to feel deeply.

So as I sit here now with the pressure of meeting the deadline on this book, I feel intense energy in the center of my heart. It feels like a tornado, the tail dipping just below my diaphragm. I've felt it since I completed my first eight-hour meditation on Christmas Eve just a few days ago, and it has now attached itself to the completion of this chapter. MB warned me of this before going so long in meditation. He said that it is possible to feel overwhelmed, anxious, or depressed after such a profound experience. And it was just that, profound. I will never be the same because I know that I touched the hand of God in that meditation.

But for every high, there is an equal low, and in the days following that meditation, my energy fell low. I felt a general malaise and overall disappointment with how we live as humans on this earth. The energy was sloth-like, slow-moving and heavy. I've talked with many athletes about the post-race blues, and this felt similar. I knew it was there to process and let go, so I started by getting curious about how I was willing to experience what I was experiencing.

I asked myself if I was willing to allow myself grace to feel so I could let go.

I asked myself if I was willing to relax when I felt impatience get its grips on me.

I asked if I was willing to walk the talk and detach from how things played out.

And if I was willing to slow down and not push through.

The answer to all was yes, and so I surrendered my attachment to the deadline. This gave me immediate relief, but I knew I had to stay ahead in the process of processing. And so I did. I kept my body moving through yoga, swimming, and walking. I journaled, meditated often, and practiced not responding to claims that time was running out. I have seen too many times how things change in an instant. In this case, four days later the skies of my mind cleared and this chapter moved through me.

On New Year's eve 2021, I was at FedEx printing out the first draft of this book. I was through it, on the other side, attained through non-resistance and detachment from what I was experiencing. The other alternative was to indulge the panic or sink into inertia. I've learned that when I feel as low and constricted as I did after that meditation, the most skillful thing to do is to allow whatever is passing through me to pass through. No fight, no resistance, no pressure, no rush.

Allowing means we release the timeline and anchor into the now moment where we can fully experience the contrast. It's the space between what we want and what we have. There is freedom in this midpoint between seeking and resisting, ease and effort. And this is where I have felt the unwanted layers do what Ram Dass said, effortlessly fall away.

Years back, I asked MB where all the energy goes that moves through me when I let go, and he told me that it transmutes back to love, the highest frequency ever measured. From this, I reasoned that each time we choose to allow *what is* over fighting *what is*, we catalyze the purification of energy back to love. Whenever we choose love over fear, kindness over judgment, or connection over separation, we vitalize higher frequencies for our life experience. By making conscious choices, we engage in mindful living, which lightens up our triggered reactions. Responding mindfully to challenges dramatically lowers stress because we are in a power position over the tendencies of our minds. With lower stress, we experience higher health. So, when I look at ideal conditions for top performance, I see meditation and mindful practices as absolute non-negotiables for better training and race execution.

Meditation also calms our nervous systems allowing our bodies to recover and our minds to quiet. It anchors us into the now moment, which is the only moment that we are available to be our best. It teaches us to watch our thoughts which heavily influence our athleticism because thoughts are things. Each one is a packet of potential, and as MB tells me, "you better have a guard at the gate." Meaning we better be watching which thoughts we are indulging because each one plants a karmic seed. And just like an acorn can only grow an oak tree, the effect of a thought can only be of the same flavor.

Researchers report that, on average, we have 60,000-70,000 thoughts per day and that 95% of those are the same thoughts we had the day before. On top of the flurry of daily repetitive thoughts, research has also found that most of our thoughts are negative and that our brains have evolved to react significantly more strongly to negative thoughts than positive ones. And even before the findings of modern-day science, Chinese philosopher and Taoist master Lao Tzu, cautioned,

"Watch your thoughts, they become your words;
watch your words, they become your actions;
watch your actions, they become your habits;
watch your habits, they become your character;
watch your character, it becomes your destiny."

If everything is energy, then that means thoughts are energy. And since beliefs are just thoughts that we think repeatedly, beliefs are energy too. And if we can transform energy, we can transform beliefs. So by training your mind to notice the present moment more, you will naturally be present to the thoughts creating your beliefs and dictating your reality.

When we are established in the now moment, change becomes available because change can only happen in the now. It is the only time we can make a change and the only time we can stay the same. Now is the only constant in this ever-changing world of circumstance. From moment to moment, cells are changing, nature is changing, and minds are changing but the present moment is timeless. There is no construct to now, nothing to capture or measure because it is and always will be now.

We need to understand and abide by clock time to function in this world, but as I learn more about myself, I see that clock time is something I allowed to be a significant factor in how I felt for a long time. And as I sat within timelessness each day and noticed the true power of now, I became curious about the roots of time, so I asked MB. I learned that farmers invented time, the Babylonians and the Egyptians, to regulate crop cycles and organize other things like community gatherings. It served as a way to navigate life logically, so we applied this mechanism throughout much of life.

Time is a navigation system that excites the data and information centers of the brain. Once a construct of the imagination, the manifestation of time lends great satisfaction to the mind because it creates the illusion of certainty. Once humans realized that clock time could regulate more than tending crops, we expanded its reach and relied more upon it.

Wake-up time, nap time, work time, leisure time, prayer time, mealtime, and bedtime. Race time, pace time, fast time, slow time, good time, and wrong time. And suppose we are not awake to our indulgence of the illusion of time, subsequent dismissal of the now and the meaning we are giving it all? Then that means we are unconsciously influencing our mood without recognizing that we are the creators of it.

How long did we sleep?

How long did we work?

How long did we meet?

How long did we walk?

How long did we swim, bike, run?

How much did we PR?

How often did we take in nutrition?

Time has become a ruler of the day, and we have allowed it also to become the ruler of us. We permit the ultimate joy sucker, *a waste of time*, and the leading stress creator, *have no time* to be major players in how we feel. As clock-time merged with the numeric system and duration merged with data, it became the time-addicted life we live today and, for athletes, a primary way to measure success.

In daily meditation, we give ourselves a break from data and information so that we can practice entering states of timelessness which is the now. Being present to the now is a muscle we must flex every day, and we must be patient in the process because, at first a sustained anchor of present-moment awareness will be near impossible. To be in pure experience independent of the commentary of your mind is a practice that you will not have mastered even after years of practicing. Still, along the way, everything in your life will get better. According to the yoga sutras, to succeed on the path of yoga, one must practice in earnest every day for a long time with sustained enthusiasm. What I have found helpful here is to list all of the reasons that I am grateful for my practice. As I focus on gratitude for my practice, gratitude for my practice expands, sustained enthusiasm persists and my life feels better. It's quite simple.

There is nothing fancy about training the mind. Any athlete accomplishing their dreams will tell you the same; the work is showing up for the work. Be relentless in your pursuit to let things go. When clinging, repeat to yourself, "let this go," and repeat that mantra until you are calm again. When you feel pressured or stressed that time is running out, relax into long, controlled exhales and question the truth of those thoughts (return to chapter six for Byron Katie's inquiry guidance) because although thoughts are real, they are not necessarily true.

As we down-regulate the nervous system by getting still and concentrating the mind, we return to our natural state of wholeness and relaxation. It is here that, over time, we identify with our inherent safety, and when we recognize our security in the now moment, we are more apt to trust and have faith in that which we cannot see. As we lean into trust and faith, we release the neediness and fear of the ego, allowing beautiful ways of being, like ahimsa and satya, to rise naturally. It is then we live in relationship with the stream of well-being that is often disregarded in this modern day. This stream is the light that shines on us all the same. The one that knows the terrible race you are about to line up for is the exact thing you need to learn what you need to learn. And the inspired dream that is coming true is ensuring you are having fun along the way. It is the light that will show you darkness as a means to grow. Soon you will not be able to unsee what you see, and the world will shift before your eyes. There are parts of you that you are blind to today, and although you may disagree, I promise you it is true. As we wake up, we open up, and as we open up, we heal the lower vibrations of our past that are still activated within us. These vibrations or samskaras affect our overall resonance and point of attraction so learning how to feel is critical to our ability to heal. Old activations will remain until we let them go, and you will grow out of every single one if you stay the course.

I recall a time when I said out loud, "I'm so glad I have nothing to work on." I had a beautiful life, a comfortable home, loving marriage, gorgeous dogs, and yet so much still to wake up to in this life. I carried darkness from this lifetime and others, brewing under the surface and contributing to the fear and doubt I accepted as a normal part of life. Living for the future and rehashing the past eventually wore on me so much that it drove me to find another way. That way was present-moment awareness through the practice of yoga. And I'm asking you to open your mind to the very same. I'm encouraging you to consider what is beneath the obvious, and I hope to invigorate you to let go of old worldviews that conjure pandemics and breed fear and doubt. I am inviting you to defy consensus thinking and be the 1% that picked up this book and stayed with it this far because you know that change begins within yourself.

The process will move faster when you release the need to know why you are a certain way. Suppose you can identify with yourself right now and move forward from here, no matter what here looks like. In that case, you will remove the drudgery caused by dragging around the dramatics of your past, and you will release yourself from the exhaustion of procrastinating life. You will face the stories that you believe justify who you are because, to become the person you came here to be, you must feel the expiration of all that you think you are now.

The cost of your new life is your old life.

I know many of you have already felt the power and shifts that come from shutting your mouth, closing your eyes, sitting down, and not moving for a series of moments each day. I know many of you have woken up during those seemingly random moments while standing in line at the grocery store or getting cut off in traffic. You acknowledge that you would be anxious or seething in the past, but instead, you take those moments to indulge in a relaxing breath. And I know many of you notice that you are listening to others now instead of waiting to be heard. So, for many of you, the awakening is already well underway. As for the rest, stay with it. I trust in the inherent power of getting to know ourselves through meditation and mindfulness, as taught through the science of the mind.

THE TIME IS NOW

I know this moment is our forever chance to begin again because the life we dream of and the athlete we desire to be, are always one choice away. We are the ones we've been waiting for; no one is coming to save us. It is already predicted that we will not see another fully enlightened being on this planet in our lifetime. It is up to us from here, and the time for our awakening is now.

Booklist

The following books were game changers for me along my
Awake Athlete path; I referenced several within the pages you
just read. I've listed them in order of how I discovered and
studied them.

The Four Agreements
by Don Miguel Ruiz

*The War Of Art: Break Through The Blocks And Win Your Creative
Battles*
by Steven Pressfield

The Bhagavad Gita
translation by Eknath Easwaran

The Untethered Soul: The Journey Beyond Yourself
by Michael Singer

The Power Of Now: A Guide To Spiritual Enlightenment
by Eckhart Tolle

Loving What Is: Four Questions The Can Change Your Life
by Byron Katie

The Yoga Sutras Of Pantanjali
by Sri Swami Satchidananda

Autobiography Of A Yogi
by Paramahansa Yogananda

The Upanishads
translation by Eknath Easwaran

The Dhammapada
translation by Eknath Easwaran

Oneness: The Teachings
by Rasha

The Yamas And Niyamas: Exploring Yoga's Ethical Practice
by Deborah Adele

The Bible
New King James version

Wishes Fulfilled: Mastering
by Dr. Wayne Dyer

The Wisdom Of Florence Scovel Schinn
by Florence Scovel Schinn

Do You Quantum Think?: New Thinking That Will Rock Your World
by Dianne Collins

The Surrender Experience: My Journey Into Life's Perfection
by Michael Singer

Bhagavad Gita As It Is
by A.C. Bhaktivedanta Swami Prabhupada

The Yoga Way: Food For Body, Mind & Spirit
by Sri Swami Satchidananda

Healing Your Life: Lessons On The Path of Ayuurveda
by Marc Halpern

The Living Gita: The Complete Bhagavad Gita — A Commentary For Modern Readers
by Sri Swami Satchidananda

Living With The Himalayan Masters
by Swami Rama

Take Your Time: The Wisdom Of Slowing Down
by Eknath Easwaran

Additional books authored by Jess Gumkowski
(Available on Amazon)

YogiTriathlete Cookbook: High Vibe Recipes for the Athlete Appetite

High Vibe Pies: Pizza Night Finally Done Right

www.ingramcontent.com/pod-product-compliance
Lightning Source LLC
Chambersburg PA
CBHW071426090426
42737CB00011B/1586